KU-712-097

Cardiac Care: An Introduction for Healthcare Professionals

WARRINGTON HOSPITAL LIBRARY

WARRINGTON HOSPITAL LIBRARY

Cardiac Care: An Introduction for Healthcare Professionals

Edited by
DAVID BARRETT, MARK GRETTON AND TOM QUINN

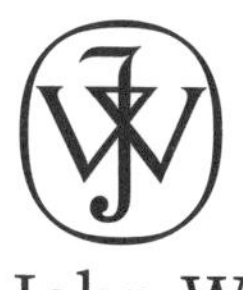

John Wiley & Sons, Ltd

WARRINGTON AND HALTON HOSPITALS
NHS FOUNDATION TRUST
B09338

Copyright © 2006 John Wiley & Sons Ltd
The Atrium, Southern Gate, Chichester,
West Sussex PO19 8SQ, England
Telephone (+44) 1243 779777

Email (for orders and customer service enquiries): cs-books@wiley.co.uk
Visit our Home Page on www.wiley.com

All Rights Reserved. No part of this publication may be reproduced, stored in a retrieval system or transmitted in any form or by any means, electronic, mechanical, photocopying, recording, scanning or otherwise, except under the terms of the Copyright, Designs and Patents Act 1988 or under the terms of a licence issued by the Copyright Licensing Agency Ltd, 90 Tottenham Court Road, London W1T 4LP, UK, without the permission in writing of the Publisher. Requests to the Publisher should be addressed to the Permissions Department, John Wiley & Sons Ltd, The Atrium, Southern Gate, Chichester, West Sussex PO19 8SQ, England, or emailed to permreq@wiley.co.uk, or faxed to (+44) 1243 770620.

Designations used by companies to distinguish their products are often claimed as trademarks. All brand names and product names used in this book are trade names, service marks, trademarks or registered trademarks of their respective owners. The Publisher is not associated with any product or vendor mentioned in this book.

This publication is designed to provide accurate and authoritative information in regard to the subject matter covered. It is sold on the understanding that the Publisher is not engaged in rendering professional services. If professional advice or other expert assistance is required, the services of a competent professional should be sought.

Other Wiley Editorial Offices

John Wiley & Sons Inc., 111 River Street, Hoboken, NJ 07030, USA

Jossey-Bass, 989 Market Street, San Francisco, CA 94103–1741, USA

Wiley-VCH Verlag GmbH, Boschstr. 12, D-69469 Weinheim, Germany

John Wiley & Sons Australia Ltd, 42 McDougall Street, Milton, Queensland 4064, Australia

John Wiley & Sons (Asia) Pte Ltd, 2 Clementi Loop #02–01, Jin Xing Distripark, Singapore 129809

John Wiley & Sons Canada Ltd, 6045 Freemont Blvd, Mississauga, ONT, L5R 4J3.

Wiley also publishes its books in a variety of electronic formats. Some content that appears in print may not be available in electronic books.

Library of Congress Cataloging-in-Publication Data

Cardiac care : an introduction for healthcare professionals/edited by
David Barrett, Mark Gretton, Tom Quinn
p. ; cm.
Includes index.
ISBN-13: 978-0-470-01983-2 (alk. paper)
ISBN-10: 0-470-01983-2 (alk. paper)
1. Heart – Diseases – Nursing. I. Barrett, David. II. Gretton, Mark. III. Quinn, Tom, 1961– .
[DNLM: 1. Heart Diseases. 2. Heart Diseases – nursing. WG 210 C2662 2006]
RC674.C25 2006
616.1′2025 – dc22

2006011820

A catalogue record for this book is available from the British Library

ISBN-13: 978-0-470-01983-2
ISBN-10: 0-470-01983-2

Printed and bound in Great Britain by TJ International Ltd, Padstow, Cornwall

This book is printed on acid-free paper responsibly manufactured from sustainable forestry in which at least two trees are planted for each one used for paper production.

Contents

Preface

People with cardiac conditions are encountered within all clinical settings. This book is written for anybody who cares for these people as part of their professional role. Although written by nurses, it is hoped that the content will be of interest and use to all health professionals.

For those healthcare professionals with little or no knowledge of cardiac disorders, it will give a basic grounding in the underlying pathophysiology of heart disease, and an understanding of available treatments. For the more experienced practitioner, the book will provide an accessible and interesting update on the latest research and trends in the fast-moving speciality of cardiac care.

The editors and contributors who have produced this book have years of experience of caring for patients with cardiac disorders. We have all seen the terrible impact of cardiac disease on patients and their families and believe passionately that the provision of holistic, evidence-based care can ease that burden.

We hope that this book will give the reader the same enthusiasm for cardiac care that we have, while also informing and educating about this fascinating speciality.

David Barrett, Mark Gretton, Tom Quinn
2006

List of contributors

David Barrett
Lecturer in Nursing, Faculty of Health and Social Care, University of Hull

Diane Burley
Senior Staff Nurse, Cardiac Intensive Care Unit, University Hospitals Coventry and Warwickshire NHS Trust

Mark Gretton
Lecturer in Nursing, Faculty of Health and Social Care, University of Hull

Joanne Hatfield
Lecturer in Nursing, Faculty of Health and Social Care, University of Hull

Tom Quinn
Professor of Cardiac Nursing and Consultant Cardiac Nurse, Faculty of Health and Life Sciences, Coventry University

Liz Smith
Lecturer in Nursing, Faculty of Health and Social Care, University of Hull

Foreword

Excellence in cardiac care is always delivered by a multi-professional team and so I was delighted to be asked to write the foreword to a book which can be so easily accessed by all health professionals in cardiac services. The authors' considerable talents and experience have made this a high quality resource. In addition, the assembled group of contributors has wide experience and is ideally placed to provide readers with good grounding and insight into the issues facing patients and their families living with heart disease.

The NHS is changing rapidly and cardiac care has seen great change, particularly since the publication of the National Service Framework for Coronary Heart Disease in March 2000. Five years later, in March 2005, a final chapter was added to fill the last gap in the patient pathway. This addressed the needs of individuals and families living with a heart rhythm problem or the consequences of having a sudden cardiac death in the family. I was delighted to see several chapters in this book covering the key issues for these patients and their families, and to see the chapter on congenital heart disease on which national guidance was published in May 2006.

The Healthcare Commission, when reviewing progress on the implementation of the National Service Framework, highlighted three areas where implementation had progressed more slowly. These were heart failure, cardiac rehabilitation and prevention. All three are addressed very well in this book. The increasing attention to primary prevention and the public health agenda has highlighted the need for health professionals to make the most of every interaction we have with patients and their families.

We know much about the determinants of heart disease and the large burden which heart disease places on our communities. We also know there are significant inequalities. This book highlights the vast amount of research in cardiac care and it will help improve care across the whole care pathway by creating a common understanding. It also reflects changes in patterns of professional education and training.

This is a timely and welcome addition to everyone's library.

Maree Barnett RN MSc MBA
Deputy Branch Head/Nurse Advisor
Vascular Programme
Department of Health

Dedication

To our parents,
Ian and Lilian Barrett,
Brenda Gretton and the late Ben Gretton, with thanks for love and support that never wavers,
Liam and Teresa Quinn, with love and thanks

1 The context of cardiac care

TOM QUINN

INTRODUCTION: THE GLOBAL BURDEN OF CARDIOVASCULAR DISEASE

Cardiovascular diseases (CVD) are the main causes of death in the modern world. According to the World Health Organization's (WHO's) *Atlas of Heart Disease and Stroke* (WHO 2004), some 17 million people die each year from CVDs, particularly as a result of acute myocardial infarction (MI) and stroke, in what is described as a 'global epidemic' (WHO 2004). Coronary heart disease (CHD) is responsible for over 7 million deaths worldwide annually. Efforts to tackle CHD in many developed countries, including the UK, are meeting with some success as a result of improvements in prevention, diagnosis and treatment. However, issues such as changing lifestyles, increasing urbanisation and longer life expectancy are responsible for an increase in the burden of CHD in developing and transitional countries. More than 60% of the global burden of CHD now occurs in developing countries and the WHO (2004) estimate that 83% of the future increases in CHD mortality will be seen in developing countries.

INTERNATIONAL COMPARISONS

The death rate from CHD in the UK has improved in recent years, but remains high relative to other developed countries, and the decline in mortality in the UK has happened at a slower pace than in other countries, e.g. in men aged 35–74 years, deaths from CHD fell by 39% between 1989 and 1999 in the UK, compared with 47% in Norway and a similar figure in Australia (British Heart Foundation or BHF 2004). For women, the corresponding figures were 41% (UK), compared with 52% (Australia), 46% (Finland) and 44% (Ireland) (BHF 2004).

Cardiac Care: An Introduction for Healthcare Professionals. Edited by David Barrett, Mark Gretton and Tom Quinn
© 2006 John Wiley & Sons Ltd

EUROPEAN STATISTICS

According to the latest European cardiovascular disease statistics published by the BHF (2005), CVD results in over 1.9 million deaths each year in the European Union (EU), and 4.35 million deaths across the continent. These data represent nearly half of all deaths in Europe and 42% of all EU deaths. CVD is the main cause of death before the age of 75 in all 15 EU countries and accounts for almost a quarter (23%) of the entire disease burden in Europe. Although death rates and incidence are falling in what might be termed 'old Europe', the countries in the north, south and west of the continent, a different pattern of slower decline or even acceleration of CVD deaths is seen in central and eastern countries of 'new Europe'.

In economic terms CVD costs the EU an estimated 169 billion Euros per annum. This can be broken down into 62% spent on health care, 21% as a result of lost productivity and 17% attributed to 'informal care' of people with CVD (BHF 2005). CVD accounted for 18% of healthcare expenditure in the UK in 2003 compared with 7% in Spain and 8% in France, against an EU average of 12% (BHF 2005).

DECLINING DEATH RATES IN THE UK

In the UK, CVD caused some 238000 deaths in 2002, almost two-fifths of all deaths that year. CHD alone accounts for 117000 deaths per annum: one in five deaths in men and one in six in women. Death rates are, however, falling – by almost half in men aged 55–64, and slightly less (40%) in men aged 35–44 during 1991–2001. In women, deaths fell by a half and a third, respectively, in age groups 55–64 and 35–44 over the same period (BHF 2004). Deaths from CVD as a whole have been steadily declining since the 1970s. The Department of Health (DH 2005b) have recently reported a 27% reduction in mortality from heart disease, stroke and related diseases since 1996 in people aged less than 75 years of age.

That death rates are declining is not, however, cause for complacency. British morbidity statistics suggest that the prevalence of CHD is on the increase in both men and women. This phenomenon seems to be particularly marked in older people (those aged 75 or more). The BHF (2004) estimate an additional 80000 people living with CHD between 2000 and 2020 as overall life expectancy increases.

Falling death rates are attributed largely to improvements in population health as well as to advances in medical care arising from both technological innovation and improved processes, ensuring more timely treatment and improved uptake of proven therapies such as cholesterol-lowering agents and aspirin. There is marked consistency in reports that treatments explain less of the decline in deaths than do changes in risk factors (Kelly and Capewell 2004). Using highly sophisticated modelling techniques, Unal et al. (2004) have been able to estimate that, compared with two decades earlier, there were some 68 230 fewer deaths resulting from CHD in England and Wales during 2000. Of these, about 26 000 were prevented by medical and surgical treatments, but the majority (36 000 or 58%) were prevented by changes in risk factors, particularly a fall in smoking prevalence. Achieving the National Service Framework for Coronary Heart Disease or NSF for CHD (DH 2000a) requirement of at least 80% of eligible patients receiving appropriate secondary prevention medication could save an additional 20 000 lives each year (Kelly and Capewell 2004). The potential impact of measures such as reduction in average cholesterol levels from 5.8 to 5.2 mmol/l would prevent around 25 000 deaths annually. Reducing smoking prevalence to rates similar to the USA could reduce deaths by 17 000 per annum. These measures, alongside small reductions in the population's blood pressure, have the potential to reduce CHD deaths by 50 000; put another way, these measures could halve the annual deaths from CHD in England and Wales.

Although the prevalence of angina, heart failure and MI is widely thought to be on the increase, the BHF (2004) have been unable to identify firm evidence to support this contention. Nevertheless, hundreds of thousands of people are living with established CHD, or will present with a new event (including MI, stroke and sudden death) each year. The burden on health services, individuals, their families and the economy remains substantial.

There are an estimated 92 000 MIs each year in men and women under 65. The BHF estimate the total number of MIs at 268 000 per annum (all ages) in the UK. Over a million survivors of MI are alive in the UK, and there are 892 000 people aged 45 years or over living with heart failure. A million people in the UK have angina pectoris (BHF 2004). Goodacre et al. (2005) have reported that 6% (700 000) of adult accident and emergency department (A&E) attendances in England and Wales annually are the result of chest pain and related complaints. Although only a minority of patients had ECG changes suggestive of an acute coronary syndrome (ACS) at presentation, two-thirds were admitted to hospital. The burden of chest pain, whether or not associated with an ACS diagnosis, on health services is therefore substantial.

REGIONAL AND SOCIOECONOMIC DIFFERENCES WITHIN THE UK

According to the BHF (2004) death rates from CHD are lowest in the south of England and highest in Scotland and the north of England. The premature death rate for men in Scotland is 50% higher than in south-west England. For women, the death rate is 90% higher. Across the UK the highest death rates from CHD are concentrated mostly in urban areas.

Although early deaths from CHD are falling across socioeconomic groups, the rate of decline is faster for non-manual workers – the BHF suggest that this means that the difference in death rates is increasing. Social inequalities in men aged 20–64 years account for the loss of an estimated 5000 lives and 47 000 working years annually. Men in manual occupations have a premature death rate 58% higher than male non-manual workers. Women in manual jobs have more than twice the rate of premature death of non-manual women. The Department of Health (2005a) state that tackling such inequalities is a high priority and that the mortality gap among people aged under 75 years has been narrowing since the late 1990s. Over this 6-year period the gap between the most deprived parts of England and the rest of the country has narrowed from 37.2 excess deaths per 100 000 population (1996–97) to 28.7 in 2001–3, a 22% reduction in the absolute gap.

People from south Asian populations in the UK have a higher than average rate of premature deaths from CHD – almost 50% higher for men and 51% for women. This difference appears to be on the increase. Premature death rates from CHD for Caribbean and west African individuals in the UK are lower than average but there are significantly higher death rates from stroke in these groups (BHF 2004).

POLICY INITIATIVES

Given the hard facts about the burden of CVD and CHD set out, it is perhaps unsurprising that reducing the incidence and mortality from CVD and CHD, and improving outcomes and experiences of people who have a CVD- or CHD-related condition, should be a high priority for governments. In post-devolution Britain, three countries have published national strategies for tackling heart disease (DH 2000a, National Assembly for Wales 2001, Scottish Executive Health Department 2002). Although each retains a distinct 'local' perspective reflecting the separate jurisdictions, there are many similarities given that each has drawn from the same international evidence base; reduction in smoking incidence, tackling blood pressure and speeding up treatment for acute events, including MI, are key features. The NSF for CHD (DH 2000a) for England has subsequently been adopted by the Spanish government (Ministerio de Sanidad Y Consumo 2001). The remainder of this chapter focuses on policies for tackling CHD in England because the author has been closely involved in their development over a number of years.

ENGLAND – THE CHD NSF

The New Labour government elected in 1997 set out its ambitions to reform the National Health Service (NHS) in a White Paper *The New NHS* (DH 1997) soon after coming to office. This was followed by *A First Class Service*

(DH 1998), which set out a programme for raising standards of NHS care including the development of NSFs for key conditions. Quality of care would be enhanced through a quality framework comprising national standards (set through NSFs and a new public authority, the National Institute for [Health and] Clinical Excellence or NICE), dependable local delivery facilitated by clinical governance, professional self-regulation and lifelong learning, and monitored by a Commission for Health Improvement, the NHS Performance Assessment Framework and the National Survey of NHS Patients. The White Paper *Saving Lives: Our healthier nation* (DH 1999) set a range of central targets for improving public health, including the following target, subsequently given the status of a high level Public Service Agreement (PSA):

> To reduce the death rate from coronary heart disease, stroke and related diseases in people under 75 by at least 40% by 2010, with at least a 40% reduction in the inequalities gap between the fifth of areas with the worst health and deprivation indicators and the population as a whole.
>
> DH (1999)

In addition the PSA target for long-term conditions encompasses services for people living with CHD, especially heart failure:

> To improve health outcomes for people with long-term conditions by offering a personalised care plan for vulnerable people most at risk and to reduce emergency bed days by 5% by 2008, through improved care in primary care and community settings for people with long-term conditions.
>
> DH (2005a)

The NSF for CHD was predicated on the evidence of inequalities in access to high-quality NHS services in England, including cardiology and cardiothoracic surgery, as well as primary and emergency care and rehabilitation. The use of effective medicines such as aspirin and statins after hospital admission with MI was inconsistent across the country. Rates of revascularisation varied according to where people lived and waiting times were excessive, with an estimated 500 deaths annually on the waiting list for bypass surgery. Despite a wealth of evidence of the time-related benefits of thrombolytic treatment in acute MI, delays were considerable and a minority of A&E departments were providing this lifesaving treatment.

The NSF for CHD, launched by the Prime Minister and Health Secretary on 6 March 2000, set out 12 national standards for improved prevention, diagnosis and care of cardiac patients to be achieved over a 10-year period. In addition, clear guidance was given to the NHS on the timescale for achievement of a range of milestones relating to, for example, the conduct of local equity audits, the development of local delivery plans, and the transfer of thrombolysis provision from cardiac care units (CCUs) to A&E departments so that 75% of the latter were able to provide this treatment. The key elements of the

Table 1.1 Summary of progress on National Service Framework delivery

Factor	Then	Now
Adult smoking prevalence (%)	28 (2000)	25 (2003)
Children receiving school fruit	0 (2000)	>2 million
Estimated lives saved by statins	2900 (2000)	9000 (2004)
Patients waiting >12 months for heart surgery	1093 (March 2000)	0 (December 2004)
Patients waiting >9 months for heart surgery	2694 (March 2000)	0 (March 2003)
Patients waiting >6 months for heart surgery	2766 (April 2002)	0 (Nov 2004)
Patients waiting >3 months for heart surgery	Expected to be 0 by end March 2005	
Percentage door to needle <30 minutes	38 (2000)	84 (December 2004)
Consultant cardiologists	467 (1999)	694 (June 2004)
Heart surgeons	182 (1999)	240 (June 2004)

Adapted from table on page 7 of *Leading the Way* (Department of Health 2005a).

NSF were reinforced in the wider-reaching NHS Plan (DH 2000b) published 3 months later. A comparison of the different health systems in the USA and the UK has been undertaken, focusing on efforts to tackle CHD (Ayanian and Quinn 2001).

The NSF for CHD was criticised on publication for being unambitious and representing nothing more than 'motherhood and apple pie . . . written at the level of a . . . medical student' (Hampton 2000). Such criticism was misplaced given that, as almost everything in the NSF for CHD had previously formed recommendations from professional societies nationally and internationally, significant variations in practice remained and the diffusion of some treatments into routine practice was patchy, a concerted effort being clearly needed to improve patient outcome and experience. Five years into its 10-year implementation process, the NSF for CHD does seem to have delivered significant improvements for patients (Table 1.1).

The focus on clearly defined 'immediate priorities', such as smoking cessation, ambulance response times and thrombolysis, rapid access chest pain clinics and waiting times for revascularisation, appears to have delivered important improvements in all these areas. However, concerns have been expressed about the lack of progress in other areas of the NSF for CHD, e.g. in services for people with heart failure and for those requiring rehabilitation (Healthcare Commission 2005). Guidance on improvements in heart failure care has been published separately (DH 2003) as has advice on addressing potential inequalities in access for Asian people with heart disease (DH 2004b). Although the key professional societies have broadly welcomed the NSF for CHD and the improvements that it has stimulated (British Cardiac Society and Royal College of Physicians 2002), continuing gaps have been highlighted in, for example, the quality of services for patients with atrial fibrillation and other arrhythmias. This last issue has been addressed in an additional NSF chapter published in March 2005 (DH 2005b), although broad 'quality requirements' have replaced the more centralist target approach, reflecting the current climate of fewer national targets.

That improvements in healthcare will require additional human resources – more cardiologists, more GPs, more nurses in a range of settings, more paramedics, clinical physiologists and many other health workers – should go without saying. Fundamental changes to the way in which these professionals work in the care of CHD patients is reflected in the variety and complexity of the competencies for CHD care published by Skills for Health (2005). The development of practitioners with special interests, based mainly in primary care, is intended further to enhance access to specialist advice for patients.

HEALTH: A MATTER OF CHOICE?

Preventing CHD is now a key priority at least equal to improvements in diagnosis and treatment, and the role of wider determinants of health in reducing CHD mortality is well established as discussed above. The recent public health White Paper *Choosing Health* (DH 2004a) set out the Government's commitment to provide more opportunities and support to help people choose to live healthier lifestyles. A range of commitments, notably to tackling health inequalities through action on smoking, nutrition and increased physical activity, were highlighted, aimed at reducing the incidence of CHD and other major conditions including diabetes, stroke and cancer. A new national target for reducing health inequalities was also announced.

Any discussion of the battle against CHD would be incomplete without emphasis on two further key elements: the important role of tobacco smoking in causing premature death, and the vital and complex function of primary care in playing a major role in supporting healthier lifestyles, identifying people at risk of developing CHD, supporting them in reducing that risk, and supporting patients and their families through recovery or long-term illness.

SMOKING

According to research commissioned by the Health Development Agency (2004) over a third of men aged under 54 and a third of women aged under 44 in England smoke. Highest rates were found among men aged 25–34 where as many as 40% were current smokers. Just over a third of adults in England were found to be ex-smokers, with differences resulting from age and geographical factors observed. Smoking was thought to be responsible for an average 86 500 deaths each year between 1998 and 2002, almost two-thirds of these deaths occurring in men. Mortality attributable to smoking is declining, with 120 000 deaths in 1995 (Health Development Agency 2004). Smoking cessation programmes were key elements of the NSF for CHD and the *Choosing Health* White Paper and a ban on smoking in enclosed public places is now on the statute books in most British countries.

THE ULTIMATE CCU? PRIMARY CARE

Primary care services in the UK have been revolutionised by the introduction of a new General Medical Services' (GMS) contract in April 2004. A key component of the GMS is a Quality and Outcomes Framework (QoF) aimed at rewarding improvements in the quality of patient care. Clinical, organisational and additional services and patient experience are four key domains assessed by a set of key indicators. Of a maximum 550 points (at the time of writing) in the clinical domain, some 356 can be gained by improvements in care for patients with CVD, diabetes or hypertension. The QoF is reliant to a large extent on computerised patient records and better use of information will enable individual practices to benchmark against other parts of the system at primary care trust, strategic health authority and national levels (Capps 2004).

CONCLUSION

Diseases of the heart and circulation are major causes of death and ill-health across the world, with the burden of disease greatest in developing countries. Major Government policies have been published across the UK to improve public health, with specific efforts aimed at better prevention, diagnosis and treatment, and expenditure in the UK on this issue is among the highest in Europe. The substantial improvements made over the past 5 years are expected to herald further advances to bring UK mortality rates nearer to those of comparable countries.

REFERENCES

Ayanian JZ, Quinn TJ (2001) Quality of care for coronary heart disease in two countries. *Health Affairs* **20**: 55–67.

British Cardiac Society and Royal College of Physicians (2002) Fifth report on the provision of services for patients with heart disease. *Heart* 88: Suppl 3:iii1–56.

British Heart Foundation (2004) *Coronary Heart Disease Statistics Database*. Available from www.heartstats.org.

British Heart Foundation (2005) *European Cardiovascular Disease Statistics*. London: BHF.

Capps N (2004) *Quality and Outcomes Framework*. Guest editorial. National Library for Health, Cardiovascular Diseases Specialist Library. Available from www.library.nhs.uk/cardiovascular.

Department of Health (1997) *The New NHS: Modern, dependable.* London: The Stationery Office.

Department of Health (1998) *A First Class Service: Quality in the new NHS*. London: Department of Health.

Department of Health (1999) *Saving Lives: Our healthier nation* London: The Stationery Office.

Department of Health (2000a) *National Service Framework for Coronary Heart Disease*. London: Department of Health.

Department of Health (2000b) *The NHS Plan*. London: The Stationery Office.

Department of Health (2003) *Developing Services for Heart Failure*. London: The Stationery Office.

Department of Health (2004a) *Choosing Health*. London: The Stationery Office.

Department of Health (2004b) *Heart Disease and South Asians*. London: The Stationery Office.

Department of Health (2005a) *Leading the Way: The coronary heart disease national service framework. Progress report 2005*. London: Department of Health.

Department of Health (2005b) *National Service Framework for Coronary Heart Disease*. Chapter 8 Arrhythmias and sudden cardiac death. London: Department of Health.

Goodacre S, Cross E, Arnold J et al. (2005) The health care burden of acute chest pain. *Heart* **91**: 229–30.

Hampton JR (2000) The National Service Framework for coronary heart disease: the emperor's new clothes. *Journal of the Royal College of Physicians of London* **34**: 226–9.

Healthcare Commission (2005) *Getting to the Heart of It. Coronary heart disease in England: A review of progress towards national standards*. London: Commission for Healthcare Audit and Inspection.

Health Development Agency (2004) *The Smoking Epidemic in England*. London: Health Development Agency.

Kelly MP, Capewell S (2004) Relative contributions of changes in risk factors and treatment to the reduction in coronary heart disease mortality. *Health Development Agency Briefing Paper*. London: Health Development Agency.

Ministerio de Sanidad Y Consumo (2001) *Enfermedad Coronaria. Plan Integral de Servicios*. Madrid: Planificacian Sanitaria.

National Assembly for Wales (2001) *Tackling CHD in Wales: Implementing through evidence*. Cardiff: Welsh Assembly Government.

Scottish Executive Health Department (2002) *Coronary Heart Disease and Stroke Strategy for Scotland*. Edinburgh: The Stationery Office.

Skills for Health (2005) *Revised Coronary Heart Disease National Workforce Competence Framework*. Available from: www.skillsforhealth.org.uk.

Unal B, Critchley JA, Capewell S (2004) Explaining the decline in coronary heart disease mortality in England and Wales between 1981 and 2000. *Circulation* **109**: 1101–7.

World Health Organization (2004) *The Atlas of Heart Disease and Stroke.* Geneva: WHO.

2 The history of cardiac care

TOM QUINN

The history of cardiac care is fascinating, and dates back thousands of years. Many of the treatments and techniques that we now take for granted have been developed over decades (and in some cases even centuries), and it is striking how the foresight of pioneering researchers and clinicians has, over time, been vindicated.

The key source for this chapter is the World Health Organization (WHO 2005) website, which provides a comprehensive history setting out a series of milestones in knowledge of heart and vascular disorders dating back to the Palaeolithic era. Although readers are encouraged to access the site in person, some of the key highlights are set out below. Very recent technological advances in equipment, techniques and therapeutics are outside the scope of the chapter. Where available, references are given at the end of the chapter; otherwise the author acknowledges the enormous value of the WHO site in providing key information.

THE FIRST DRAWING OF A HEART

The oldest drawing of a heart is thought to be from the Palaeolithic era; a cave in El Pindal, Spain has a drawing of a mammoth on the wall, with a dark smudge at the shoulder thought to represent the heart.

DESCRIBING THE CIRCULATION

The first description of circulatory flow is thought to be contained in the *Nei Ching* (*Canon of Medicine*) dating back to 2968–2598 BC. The Chinese Yellow Emperor, Huang Ti, wrote: 'The blood current flows continuously in a circle without a beginning or an end and never stops . . . all the blood is under control of the heart.'

In early Egypt, Erasistratus (310–250 BC) described the circulatory system, including valves, but suggested that the arteries carried 'pneuma' (air), replaced with every breath. When an artery was cut, blood rushed in as pneuma escaped.

Cardiac Care: An Introduction for Healthcare Professionals. Edited by David Barrett, Mark Gretton and Tom Quinn
© 2006 John Wiley & Sons Ltd

The liver was thought for many years (by, for example the Roman physician Claudius Galen [AD 131–201] and Leonardo da Vinci [1452–1519]) to be the centre of the circulation. This was refuted by Andreas Vesalius in 1555. The first use in modern times of the term 'blood circulation' was by the Italian Andrea Cesalpino (1525–1603). The presence of two main coronary arteries was first described by Riva di Trento in 1559. William Harvey, an English physician, published his thesis that the heart pumped blood around the body in *De Motu Cordis* in 1628.

BLOOD PRESSURE

Blood pressure was first measured by an English clergyman, Stephen Hales, who reported in 1733 an experiment in which he inserted a brass tube into the artery of a horse to demonstrate the pressure exerted by the heart to pump blood. The sphygmomanometer was subsequently invented in 1896 by Scipione Riva-Rocci. Hypertension was identified as a treatable risk factor for stroke in the 1960s and the value of lowering blood pressure to prevent coronary disease was confirmed by meta-analysis in 1990.

ANGINA PECTORIS

The link between angina pectoris and coronary heart disease was made by Edward Jenner (1749–1832), best known for his discovery of smallpox vaccine. Angina was described by William Heberden in 1772 with the classic description:

> They who are afflicted, are seized while they are walking (especially . . . uphill and soon after eating) with a painful and most disagreeable sensation in the breast, which seems as if it would extinguish life if it were to increase or continue; but the moment they stand still, all this uneasiness vanishes.

Lauder Brunton described the use of amyl nitrate to relieve angina symptoms in 1867. The first use of exercise as a test to provoke angina was reported by the Americans Charles Wolferth and Francis Wood in 1931.

LIPIDS

Heberden is also given credit for the first description of hyperlipidaemia when he wrote that the serum of a patient who had died suddenly was 'thick like cream'. The term 'cholesterol' was later coined by the Frenchman Chevreul in 1815, whose compatriot Louis Rene Lecanu showed, in 1838, that cholesterol was present in human blood. Sir Richard Quain related the presence of fatty materials in coronary arteries to nutrition in 1852. The correlation between mortality risk and cholesterol levels was demonstrated along with numerous other risk factors – including smoking and hypertension – by the Framingham study in the 1960s (Kannel et al. 1961) and 1970s, and confirmed in the 1980s. In later years Nobel Prizes for Medicine would be awarded to Konrad Bloch and Feodor Lynen in 1964 for their work on metabolism of cholesterol and fatty acids, and to Michael Brown and Joseph Goldstein in 1985 for their discovery of the low-density lipoprotein (LDL) pathway. The earliest statin, compactin, was discovered by Akiro Endo in Japan in 1976 (Endo 1992, Mehta and Khan 2002).

DIGOXIN AND ATRIAL FIBRILLATION

In 1785 the West Midlands physician William Withering described the use of digitalis (foxglove) in heart disease. Atrial fibrillation (AF) was first reported by Arthur Cushney in 1907. The additional risk of stroke associated with AF was not recognised, however, until the late 1970s.

SOUNDING AND VIEWING THE HEART

The stethoscope was invented by Rene Theophile Laennee in 1819, possibly on the grounds of chivalry: he was reluctant to apply his ear to the chest of a young woman patient and instead used paper rolled into a cylinder to avoid physical contact. Echocardiography was pioneered by the Swedes Inge Edler and Hellmuth Hertz (who also invented the ink-jet printer), building on sonar technology developed to detect submarines in World War II (Edler and Hertz 1954).

DEFIBRILLATION

Ventricular fibrillation (VF) was first described in 1850. The history of the development of the widely used technique of defibrillation is worth retelling at some length.

The first report of complete recovery from VF treated by electrical defibrillation in humans was published by Beck et al. (1947). A 14-year-old boy had undergone an operation to correct a congenital defect. At the end of the operation the boy collapsed, apparently dead. His chest was reopened and direct cardiac massage instigated. The ECG demonstrated VF. After about 45 minutes of direct cardiac massage and artificial ventilation, an electric shock was applied directly to the heart, without success. A further series of shocks, however, resulted in resumption of cardiac activity. Three hours after the event, the boy was reported to be responding rationally to questioning, and at 8 hours was 'fairly alert'. The patient was discharged home 25 days later, and was reported at 3-month follow-up to be well, with a 'considerable increase' in exercise tolerance, and without detectable neurological or cardiac damage (Beck et al. 1947).

The first successful defibrillation of a patient with myocardial infarction (MI) was reported by Reagan et al. (1956). A 55-year-old truck driver presented with chest pain, and developed VF during the recording of an ECG in the emergency room. His chest was opened almost immediately and, after a period of 15 minutes, the heart was defibrillated. The patient made a full recovery and was reported to be back at full-time work 8 months later (Reagan et al. 1956).

Working independently, Beck et al. (1956) described the successful defibrillation of a 65-year-old physician, who had presented to hospital with chest pain. The diagnosis of early posterolateral MI was made on the basis of an initial ECG. Ninety minutes later, the patient collapsed while leaving the hospital (the reason for this somewhat premature discharge from hospital is not recorded). His chest was opened within 4 minutes, and the heart shocked after 5 minutes of direct cardiac massage, without success. Resuscitation continued for 30 minutes, and the patient ultimately recovered sufficiently to resume his medical practice.

In reporting their historic achievement (acknowledging that Reagan et al. had been the first to succeed), Beck's team suggested that trained resuscitation teams be made available in hospitals to respond immediately to sudden death from heart attack, and that steps be taken to teach cardiopulmonary resuscitation (CPR) to laypeople for use in the community setting:

> The veil of mystery is being lifted from heart conditions, and the dead are being brought back to life.
>
> Beck et al. (1956)

THE CORONARY CARE UNIT

The history of coronary care is linked closely to that of CPR. The concept of a specialised ward dedicated to the observation, care and resuscitation of patients with acute MI or ischaemia was first proposed by a British cardiologist, Desmond Julian, in 1961. Patients across the world have benefited from 'cardiac care units' for over 40 years as a result of Julian's (1961) vision.

PACEMAKERS

External countershock to terminate VF was first reported in 1956 by Zoll (Zoll et al. 1956). He also designed the external cardiac pacemaker in 1952 (building on Hyman's earlier [1932] work using a transthoracic needle to stimulate the heart), although the first pacemaker is said to have been invented by the Canadian, John Hopps, in 1950. In 1958 a patient survived for 96 days after insertion of a pacemaker by Seymour Furman. Ake Senning introduced long-term internal cardiac pacing in 1958 in Sweden (Elmqvist 1978).

THE ELECTROCARDIOGRAM

Rudolf von Koelliker and Heinrich Muller discovered, in 1856, that the heart generated electricity (Bursch and DePasquale 1964). Muirhead achieved the first recording of electrical rhythm from a human heart in 1869 at St Bartholomew's Hospital in London. Augustus Waller coined the term 'cardiograph' in 1887 when he published the first report of a recording of cardiac electricity on the body surface. He went on to present preliminary data on 2000 electrocardiograms at a meeting of the Physiological Society of London in 1917 (Waller 1917). Waller was not initially convinced of the potential of his new technique, saying:

> I do not imagine that electrocardiography is likely to find any very extensive use in the hospital. It can be of rare and occasional use to afford a record of some rare anomaly of cardiac action.
>
> Barker (1910)

William Einthoven (1860–1927), who introduced the term electrocardiogram (ECG) in 1893, described the PQRST deflections in 1895, and built the first ECG machine (weighing 270 kg) in 1901, had been in the audience at a presentation given by Waller in London during 1887. Einthoven transmitted the first ECG in 1905, published normal and abnormal ECGs in 1906 and was awarded the Nobel Prize in 1924. The first ECG showing acute MI was reported in the USA by Harold Pardee in 1920. Holter developed the first ambulatory ECG monitor in 1949. Interpretation of the ECG was standardised with the introduction of the Minnesota Code (Blackburn 1969).

ASPIRIN

Aspirin was introduced in 1897 but the Bayer advertisements of the time reassured the public that the drug did 'not affect the heart'. In 1948, Lawrence Craven described how 400 of his male patients who took aspirin for 2 years avoided heart attacks. He observed a larger cohort of 8000 patients taking aspirin, reporting in 1956 that people taking this treatment suffered no heart attacks. Aspirin's role in cardiovascular disease prevention became more widely accepted in the 1970s and the lifesaving potential of this widely available drug in the treatment of acute MI became widely known after the publication of the ISIS-2 (Second International Study of Infarct Survival) thrombolytic trial in 1988.

CARDIAC CATHETERISATION AND ANGIOPLASTY

Bleichroeder, Unger and Loeb, in 1912, performed the first human cardiac catheterisation, without radiographs. In Germany, Forssmann used radiological techniques to perform the first right heart catheterisation in 1929. Mason

Sones began to develop a more selective coronary angiography procedure in 1958 (Sones and Shirley 1962). Charles T. Dotter performed the first transluminal angioplasty on a narrowed vessel in 1964 (Dotter and Judkins 1964). The first percutaneous transluminal coronary angioplasty (PTCA) was performed by Andreas Gruntzig in Switzerland in 1977, successfully restoring blood flow to a blocked coronary artery (Hurst 1986). Rentrop et al. (1979) described the early experience of acute MI angioplasty 2 years later. The first intracoronary stent was implanted by Jacques Puel and Ulrich Sigwart in France in 1986 (Sigwart et al. 1987).

CARDIAC SURGERY

The first human open heart operation was performed by John Heysham Gibbon in 1953 using the prototype heart–lung machine that he developed in 1937 (Gibbon 1978). The first human heart surgery – closure of a patent ductus arteriosus – was performed by Robert E. Gross in 1938. In 1944, Crafoord and Grosse reported, from Sweden, the first repair of coarctation of the aorta. The first prosthetic aortic valve was implanted by Charles Hufnagel (USA) in 1952. The first mitral valve replacement was reported by Judson Chesterman (UK) in 1955. Albert Starr and Lowell Edwards developed the Starr–Edwards valve in 1960. Michael DeBakey and Adrian Kantrowitz pioneered the use of implanted devices to support failing hearts in 1965. In 1967, Christiaan Barnard, a South African, performed the first human heart transplantation. Rene Favoloro in the USA introduced saphenous vein coronary bypass grafting in the same year. Denton Cooley implanted the first artificial heart for human use in 1969. The first permanent artificial heart was designed by Robert Jarvik and implanted by Willem DeVries in 1982.

THROMBOLYTIC THERAPY

There are salutary lessons to be learned about how to conduct, report and interpret clinical trials so that patients can begin to benefit at the earliest (safe) opportunity – the history of thrombolytic treatment is a clear example of how a treatment can be 'proven' but under-utilised for decades because of a lack of understanding of the evidence base. It is noteworthy that randomisation of patients into clinical trials to minimise bias in the assessment of cardiovascular treatments was pioneered by Sir Austin Bradford Hill in the UK in the 1950s. The large-scale 'megatrials' with which we are now so familiar were introduced at the instigation of the British scientist Sir Richard Peto in the 1980s.

Fletcher et al. first described the feasibility of treating acute MI patients with thrombolytic therapy to disperse thrombus and limit infarct size in 1958. Thrombolytic therapy did not, however, become routine treatment for MI until the late 1980s.

This delay in implementation probably cost hundreds of thousands of lives worldwide. Despite Herrick's (1912) earlier observations, the belief persisted for many years that 'coronary thrombosis' was a secondary, rather than a primary, responsible event. The primary role of thrombus was demonstrated convincingly by De Wood et al. as late as 1980. In the 20 years after Fletcher et al.'s (1958) observations, a number of studies were undertaken, but, of the 33 trials comparing intravenous streptokinase with placebo or no therapy reported between 1959 and 1988, statistically significant benefit was seen in only six (Lau et al. 1992). Lau et al.'s (1992) meta-analysis of these trials significantly favoured treatment, leading Mulrow (1995) to conclude that intravenous streptokinase 'could have been shown to be life saving almost 20 years ago'.

The key trials in establishing thrombolysis as a mainstream treatment for acute MI were reported in the late 1980s – GISSI-1 (1986) and ISIS-2 (1988). A collaborative overview of nine large, randomised trials of thrombolysis (Fibrinolytic Therapy Trialists' [FTT] Collaborative Group 1994), including GISSI-1 and ISIS-2, and involving some 58 600 patients, demonstrated highly significant mortality reduction with thrombolytic treatment: 30 per 1000 patients for those treated within 6 hours of symptom onset, and 20 per 1000 for those treated within 7–12 hours. Boersma et al. (1996) presented an alternative analysis of the importance of very early thrombolysis in support of the concept of a 'first golden hour' in which a substantial additional reduction in mortality is achievable. Benefits of very early treatment appear striking: 65 lives saved per 1000 patients treated in the first hour from symptom onset, 37 in hours 1–2 and 29 in hours 2–3. Proportional mortality reduction was significantly higher in those treated within 2 hours compared with those treated later. Such observations have prompted efforts to provide thrombolysis at the earliest opportunity, including in the pre-hospital phase of care, as discussed in Chapter 7.

CONCLUSION

As stated in the introduction to this chapter, the history of cardiac care is indeed fascinating. One can only speculate about what advances lie in the future, with stem cell and other research being highly promising. Whether 'winning the war on heart disease' will rely on development of breakthrough medicines, genetics, or interventional and surgical techniques, or in renewed efforts to implement the evidence that we have on what works, or in tackling the wider determinants of health through improved public health measures, remains a matter for debate and for the attention of future historians. There is no doubt, however, that cardiovascular care is an exciting area in which to practise and do research.

REFERENCES

Barker LF (1910) Electrocardiography and phonocardiography: a collective review. *Bulletin of the Johns Hopkins Hospital* **21**: 358–89.

Beck CS, Pritchard WH, Feil HS (1947) Ventricular fibrillation of long duration abolished by electric shock. *Journal of the American Medical Association* **135**: 985–6.

Beck CS, Weckesser EC, Barry FM (1956) Fatal heart attack and defibrillation. *Journal of the American Medical Association* **161**: 434–6.

Blackburn H (1969) Classification of the electrocardiogram for population studies: the Minnesota Code. *Journal of Electrocardiology* **2**: 305–10.

Boersma E, Maas ACP, Deckers JW, Simoons ML (1996) Early thrombolytic treatment in acute myocardial infarction: reappraisal of the golden hour. *Lancet* **348**: 771–5.

Bursch GE, DePasquale NP (1964) *A History of Electrocardiography*. Chicago: Year Book Medical Publishers.

De Wood MA, Spores J, Notske R et al. (1980) Prevalence of total coronary occlusion during the early hours of transmural myocardial infarction. *New England Journal of Medicine* **303**: 897–902.

Dotter CT, Judkins MP (1964) Transluminal treatment of an arteriosclerotic obstruction: description of a new technic and a preliminary report of its application. *Circulation* **30**: 654–70.

Edler I, Hertz CH (1954) Use of ultrasonic reflectoscope for the continuous recording of movement of heart walls. *Kungl Fysiogr Sallsk Lund Forh* **24**: 40.

Elmqvist R (1978) Review of early pacemaker development. *Pacing and Clinical Electrophysiology* **1**: 535–6.

Endo A (1992) The discovery and development of HMG-CoA inhibitors. *Journal of Lipid Research* **33**: 1569–82.

Fibrinolytic Therapy Trialists' (FTT) Collaborative Group (1994) Indications for fibrinolytic therapy in suspected acute myocardial infarction: collaborative overview of early mortality and major morbidity results from all randomised trials of more than 1000 patients. *Lancet* **343**: 311–22.

Fletcher AP, Alkjaersig N, Smyrniotis FE, Sherry S (1958) The treatment of patients suffering from early myocardial infarction with massive and prolonged streptokinase therapy. *Transcripts of the Association of American Physicians* **71**: 287–96.

Gibbon JH Jr (1978) The development of the heart-lung apparatus. *American Journal of Surgery* **135**: 608–19.

Gruppo Italiano per lo Studio della Streptochinasi nell' Infarcto Miocardio (GISSI) (1986) Effectiveness of intravenous thrombolytic therapy in acute myocardial infarction. *Lancet* **i**: 397–412.

Heberden W (1772) Some account of a disorder of the breast. *Medical Transcripts of the College of Physicians* **2**: 59.

Herrick JB (1912) Clinical features of sudden obstruction of coronary arteries. *Journal of the American Medical Association* **59**: 2015–20.

Hurst JW (1986) The first coronary angioplasty as described by Andreas Gruentzig. *American Journal of Cardiology* **57**: 185–6.

Hyman AS (1932) Resuscitation of the stopped heart by intracardial therapy. *Archives of Internal Medicine* **50**: 283–305.

ISIS-2 (Second International Study of Infarct Survival) Collaborative Group (1988) Randomised trial of intravenous streptokinase, oral aspirin, both, or neither among 17 187 cases of suspected acute myocardial infarction: ISIS-2. *Lancet* **ii**: 349–60.

Julian DG (1961) Treatment of cardiac arrest in acute myocardial ischaemia and infarction. *Lancet* **ii**: 840–4.

Kannel WB, Dawber TR, Kagan A et al. (1961) Factors of risk in the development of coronary heart disease – six year follow-up experience. The Framingham Study. *Annals of Internal Medicine* **55**: 33–50.

Lau J, Antman EM, Jimenez-Silva J et al (1992) Cumulative meta-analysis of therapeutic trials for myocardial infarction. *New England Journal of Medicine* **327**: 248–54.

Mehta NJ, Khan IA (2002) Cardiology's 10 greatest discoveries of the 20th Century. *Texas Heart Institute Journal* **29**: 164–71.

Mulrow CD (1995) Rationale for systematic reviews. In: Chalmers I, Altman DG (eds), *Systematic Reviews*. London: BMJ Publishing Group, pp 1–8.

Reagan LB, Young KR, Nicholson JW (1956) Ventricular defibrillation in a patient with probable acute coronary occlusion. *Surgery* **39**: 482–6.

Rentrop KP, Blanke H, Karsch KR, Kreuzer H (1979) Initial experience with transluminal recanalization of the recently occluded infarct-related coronary artery in acute myocardial infarction – comparison with conventionally treated patients. *Clinical Cardiology* **2**: 92–105.

Sigwart U, Puel J, Mirkovitch V et al. (1987) Intravascular stents to prevent occlusion and restenosis after transluminal angioplasty. *New England Journal of Medicine* **316**: 701–6.

Sones FM Jr, Shirley EK (1962) Cine coronary arteriography. *Modern Concepts of Cardiovascular Disease* **31**: 735–8.

Waller AD (1917) A preliminary survey of 2000 electrocardiograms. Proceedings of the Physiological Society, July 28, 1917. *Journal of Physiology* **51**: xvii–xviii.

World Health Organization (2005) *Milestones in Knowledge of Heart and Vascular Disorders*. Available from: www.who.int/cardiovascular_diseases/resources/atlas/en/index.html.

Zoll PM, Linenthal AJ, Gibson W, Paul MH, Norman LR (1956) termination of ventricular fibrillation in man by externally applied electric countershock. *New England Journal of Medicine* **254**: 727–32.

3 Disease prevention and rehabilitation

DAVID BARRETT

The declining death rate from coronary heart disease (CHD) in the UK over previous years has been discussed in Chapter 1. This chapter seeks to discuss two important factors underpinning this decline in mortality: disease prevention and cardiac rehabilitation.

It is important to clarify some key terms related to this topic, notably primary and secondary prevention. Primary prevention refers to interventions designed to educate and modify risk factors in individuals who have not yet been diagnosed with CHD, to reduce the likelihood of disease developing (American Heart Association 1997). Secondary prevention involves similar interventions, but focused on individuals who have established disease, with the goal of reducing the risk of further disease progression and cardiac events (Hobbs 2004).

The first part of the chapter summarises the key risk factors related to the development of heart disease, and outlines possible treatment strategies. The second part discusses specific assessment and treatment plans related to risk stratification, primary and secondary prevention, and cardiac rehabilitation.

RISK FACTORS AND MANAGEMENT STRATEGIES

SMOKING

Although rates have decreased significantly in the last 30 years, 28% of men and 25% of women within the UK still smoke (British Heart Foundation or BHF 2005). Smoking still remains a significant causative factor in many common causes of death, such as lung cancer and chronic obstructive pulmonary disease. In terms of cardiovascular disease, smoking is responsible for as many as one in five premature deaths in the UK – about 31 000 per year (BHF 2005).

Smoking contributes to the development of CHD through a number of direct and indirect mechanisms. These include damaging the endothelium of

Cardiac Care: An Introduction for Healthcare Professionals. Edited by David Barrett, Mark Gretton and Tom Quinn
© 2006 John Wiley & Sons Ltd

coronary arteries, increasing the risk of chronic hypertension and promoting the formation of thrombi (Gordon and Libby 2003). The benefits of giving up smoking are significant. Within 2 years of stopping smoking, the risk of a coronary event has halved. After between 5 and 15 years of quitting, the risk of a cardiac problem is the same as for someone who has never smoked (Gaziano et al. 2005).

Support for smoking cessation

Smoking cessation is a key element in the UK Government's policy on the primary prevention of CHD and is a priority for all patients with pre-existing CHD (Health Development Agency or HDA 2001, Dalal et al. 2004). In the UK, smoking cessation services have been heavily invested in since the publication of the National Service Framework for Coronary Heart Disease (NSF for CHD). Within that document, a support structure for smoking cessation was advocated, with services particularly focused on those patients with CHD and those at high risk of developing the disease (Department of Health or DH 2000).

Education and counselling for patients can be provided in isolation or in partnership with self-help programmes. However, without additional pharmacological intervention, the 1-year success rates for smoking cessation are as low as 10–20% (National Institute for [Health and] Clinical Excellence or NICE 2002a, Gaziano et al. 2005).

Nicotine replacement therapy (NRT) has become an important element in many smoking cessation programmes. Nicotine patches, gum and lozenges are examples of delivery systems for nicotine replacement that can complement psychological support by reducing cravings and symptoms of withdrawal (NICE 2002a). Recently, a pharmacological agent called bupropion (Zyban) has been introduced as an alternative to NRT. Unlike NRT, which provides the patient with a small level of nicotine from sources other than smoking, bupropion acts directly to reduce the craving for nicotine (NICE 2002a).

DIET

Dyslipidaemia

Dyslipidaemia is a term referring to abnormalities in the level of fats within the blood, usually resulting from genetic or lifestyle factors (Thompson 2004). Much of the emphasis related to lipid levels is focused on cholesterol, a type of lipid that is carried around the body within substances called lipoproteins. In relation to CHD risk, two lipoproteins are of particular interest – high-density lipoprotein (HDL) and low-density lipoprotein (LDL) (Gaw and Shepherd 2004).

In healthy people, the target figure for total plasma cholesterol levels is <5.0 mmol/l, although about two-thirds of the adult population in the UK have a total cholesterol level above this (BHF 2005). High levels of total plasma cholesterol have been shown to correlate closely with the risk of CHD. Some studies have suggested that a 10% increase in total serum cholesterol is associated with up to a 30% increase in CHD risk (Gaziano et al. 2005). More specifically, it is raised LDL-cholesterol levels that are closely linked to a propensity for atherosclerotic plaques to form and for CHD to develop. Whereas a high level of LDL-cholesterol is a risk factor for CHD, HDL-cholesterol actually appears to protect against the disease (Hatchett and Thompson 2002). Interventions targeted at cholesterol levels, whether related to primary or to secondary prevention, therefore strive towards lowering plasma LDL concentrations, while raising HDL-cholesterol levels.

When assessing lipid levels, account should also be taken of the triglyceride level – triglyceride is a type of lipid found within the bloodstream. Increased levels of triglycerides (>1.5 mmol/l) have been identified as increasing the likelihood of CHD, both as an independent risk factor and through causing abnormalities in LDL and HDL levels (Griffin and Whitehead 2004, Hobbs 2004).

As with smoking cessation, management of lipid levels can be achieved using two strategies: education/support and pharmacological adjuncts. Education about the level and type of fats in food is important for the population as a whole, but particularly so for those patients with, or at risk of developing, CHD. The NSF for CHD outlines how simple steps such as reducing saturated fat intake (e.g. butter and red meat), and increasing the intake of fresh fruit and vegetables should be advocated to the population as a whole (Health Development Agency 2001). Recently, the intake of plant sterols within the diet has gained popularity and publicity as a means of reducing cholesterol levels. Plant sterols are now used as an additive in a number of margarines, yoghurts and health drinks, with some evidence to suggest that regular intake can significantly reduce LDL-cholesterol levels (Thompson 2004).

Pharmacological management of raised cholesterol levels has become a crucial element in the primary and secondary prevention of CHD since the introduction of statins in the 1990s. A fuller discussion of the pharmacological actions and clinical benefits of statins can be found in Chapter 13. Since their introduction, the use of lipid-lowering drugs has increased rapidly, and the NHS now spends more money on this class of drug than on any other (BHF 2005).

In terms of primary prevention, patients with high cholesterol levels who are deemed at risk of developing CHD, and in whom lifestyle changes have not been sufficient, should be placed on a statin (Gaw and Shepherd 2004). All patients with existing CHD, particularly those who have had a myocardial infarction (MI), should also receive a statin in addition to individualised dietary advice (DH 2000, NICE 2006).

Obesity

Although obesity is being discussed in the context of dietary risk factors, the causes and effects of obesity are multidimensional. The definition of obesity is based on a calculation of the patient's body mass index (BMI), which can be made by dividing the patient's weight in kilograms by the square of their height in metres (i.e. $BMI = [weight (kg)]/[height (m)]^2$). A patient is deemed overweight if the BMI is >25, whereas a BMI >30 represents obesity. Although the BMI accounts for a patient's weight and height, it gives no indication of where excess body fat is distributed. The risk of CHD is greater if fat deposits are central (i.e. around the waist area). For this reason, BMI calculation should be accompanied by a record of the circumference of the patient's waist, with figures of 102 cm for males and 88 cm for females being regarded as the upper limit of normal (Griffin and Whitehead 2004). Fat distribution can also be evaluated through calculating the patient's waist: hip ratio, which should be <0.95 in men and <0.85 in women (BHF 2005). Patients displaying excessive waist circumference or waist:hip ratio are classed as centrally obese.

Rates of obesity within the UK have been rapidly increasing over recent years. Currently over one-fifth of men and women are classed as obese (BMI > 30), and almost one-third of adults meet the criteria for central obesity (BHF 2005). Obesity is linked to a wide range of healthcare problems, including CHD. Much of the relationship between CHD and obesity is the result of an increased prevalence of additional risk factors in obese people – notably hypertension, dyslipidaemia and type 2 diabetes.

Interventions to tackle obesity will usually run parallel to other strategies to lower the risk of CHD. In particular, patients will often enter into an individualised programme of dietary restriction and increase in physical activity. In those patients for whom changes to diet and levels of activity are not reducing weight to an acceptable level, pharmacological intervention is an option. Two drug therapies, orlistat and sibutramine, are currently licensed for use in obese patients in the UK. Orlistat works by reducing the ability of the body to absorb fat, whereas sibutramine acts on receptors in the brain to inhibit appetite (NICE 2001a, 2001b).

For patients in whom lifestyle modification and drug therapy have failed, there are two main surgical options. Restrictive operations such as gastroplasty (sometimes referred to as 'stomach stapling') physically reduce the amount of food that the patient can take in. Other operations, such as biliopancreatic diversion, do restrict the amount of food that can be eaten, but primarily work by bypassing areas of the small intestine, thereby reducing the body's ability to absorb fat (NICE 2002b). Although weight loss surgery is relatively rare within the UK, rates are increasing. Between 2004 and 2005, the number of surgical procedures performed to enhance weight loss doubled to over 4000 (British Obesity Surgery Patient Association 2005).

Alcohol

Moderate levels of alcohol consumption have been linked with a significant reduction in the likelihood of CHD (Thompson and Webster 2004). More specifically, mild-to-moderate consumption of wine provides additional decrease in risk of CHD in comparison to other alcoholic drinks (Grønbaek 2004). However, alcohol consumption beyond the current recommended guidelines of 2–3 units/day for women and 3–4 units/day for men is related to an increased risk of CHD (Griffin and Whitehead 2004).

ACTIVITY LEVELS

Regular physical activity reduces the risk of heart disease. A sedentary lifestyle increases the chances of developing two major risk factors for heart disease – obesity and type 2 diabetes – and is also an independent risk factor. Adults with an inactive lifestyle generally have twice the risk of dying from CHD as fit and active people (DH 2004). Healthy adults with no history of CHD should be encouraged, as a minimum, to undertake moderate physical activity, for at least 30 minutes, five times a week (DH 2004). Patients with established CHD should have their activity levels carefully established on the basis of an individual clinical assessment (European Society of Cardiology or ESC 2003).

HYPERTENSION

Hypertension, or high blood pressure, is closely linked to an increased risk of heart disease (Maron et al. 2004). Although optimal blood pressure is defined as <120/80 mmHg, medical intervention to reduce blood pressure (BP) is indicated only when systolic BP ≥140 mmHg and/or diastolic BP ≥90 mmHg (ESC 2003). Within the UK, almost a third of men and women meet this criterion, although the majority of these people are not receiving any treatment (BHF 2005).

Treatment options will vary depending on the severity of hypertension and overall risk of CHD. For otherwise healthy patients with a small risk of developing CHD, mild hypertension (systolic BP 140–159 mmHg, diastolic BP 90–99mmHg) can be treated through lifestyle advice. The main changes that should be encouraged to reduce BP are reduction in body weight (in overweight or obese patients), increased levels of physical activity, smoking cessation, and reduction in salt and alcohol consumption to the recommended levels (Williams et al. 2004). If lifestyle advice does not result in a decrease in BP to <140/90 mmHg, then drug treatment may be an option, particularly if the patient is deemed at risk of cardiovascular disease. Any patient in whom BP is sustained >160/100 mmHg (moderate hypertension) despite lifestyle changes should be treated pharmacologically (Williams et al. 2004). It should be noted that any patients presenting with severe hypertension

(BP ≥ 180/110 mmHg) should be treated promptly with a combination of drug therapy and lifestyle advice.

A number of drug types are used in the treatment of hypertension: β blockers, angiotensin-converting enzyme (ACE) inhibitors, calcium channel blockers, angiotensin II receptor blockers and diuretics. Details of these types of drug, including uses and side effects, are given in Chapter 13. Although drug treatment will often start with just one of these therapies, many patients will require a combination of two or three drugs to control BP adequately (ESC 2003).

The threshold for pharmacological treatment of hypertension is much lower in patients who are deemed at high risk of developing CHD. Patients within this category will often need drug therapy for treatment of mild hypertension. In some cases, such as in patients with established CHD or diabetes, antihypertensive treatment (lifestyle advice ± drug therapy) is indicated at even lower levels (≥130/80 mmHg).

DIABETES

People with diabetes are at significantly higher risk of developing heart disease than non-diabetic members of the population. Of the 1.9 million people diagnosed with diabetes in the UK, about 90% have type 2 diabetes, a condition that can increase the risk of CHD by as much as five times (BHF 2005). This large increase in CHD risk is in part a direct result of the condition, and also of the fact that diabetes magnifies the effects of other risk factors, such as hypertension, dyslipidaemia and obesity (BHF 2005). Although diabetes is not curable, good control of glucose levels is encouraged as a means to slow or prevent the development of heart disease (ESC 2003). In type 1 diabetes (usually controlled by insulin injection), insulin dosage and dietary intake should be closely controlled. In type 2 diabetes, which is usually controlled without the need for insulin injections, the focus should be on offering advice and support to control glucose and cholesterol levels, lose weight, reduce BP and increase physical activity (ESC 2003, Gibson 2003).

AGE, FAMILY HISTORY, SOCIOECONOMIC STATUS, GENDER AND ETHNICITY

Age is one of the most important risk factors for CHD. The older an individual is, the more likely it is that he or she will develop heart disease (Maron et al. 2004). The effect of gender on rates of heart disease is particularly significant in members of the population aged <55 years, with men being much more likely to develop CHD. It is hypothesised that hormones (notably oestrogen) present within premenopausal women reduce CHD risk. This suggestion is supported by figures that demonstrate a rapid increase in CHD rates in women over the age of 55 (Lindsay 2004, Maron et al. 2004).

Any person with a parent or sibling who develops CHD prematurely (≤55 in men, ≤65 in women) is viewed as having a positive family history (Maron et al. 2004). Any individual with a positive family history is him- or herself at greater risk of developing CHD and should be carefully screened for other risk factors.

There are wide variations in rates of heart disease depending on ethnic background. Adults living in the UK with a south Asian background (i.e. from India, Pakistan, Sri Lanka or Bangladesh) have significantly higher rates of morbidity and mortality from CHD than average. Conversely, adults with a Caribbean or West African background have lower rates of CHD than average (BHF 2005).

In relation to socioeconomic status, there is a documented link between low income and increased risk of heart disease within developed countries. Although the exact mechanisms for this are unclear, the links between socioeconomic status and CHD may relate to levels of stress, lifestyle choices and differences in the ability to access healthcare (World Health Organization or WHO 2004)

RISK ASSESSMENT AND PROGRAMMES FOR PREVENTION

PRIMARY PREVENTION

The risks of developing heart disease can be minimised using two broad strategies. The first is to try to reduce the prevalence of heart disease within the entire population. National policies with this aim are discussed to some degree in Chapter 1. Broadly speaking, the thrust of policy is to encourage widespread risk factor modification through promotion of healthy eating, smoking cessation, moderate alcohol intake and increased physical activity (HDA 2001).

The second important element of primary prevention is identifying and supporting those individuals at high risk of developing heart disease, a process requiring a systematic and validated risk assessment. Risk assessment for CHD is often complicated by the fact that the risk factors discussed above rarely appear in isolation, e.g. an adult who is obese may also be hypertensive and lead a sedentary life. A number of models for CHD risk estimation have been developed. One such scoring system, recently developed and recommended for use within the UK, is the Joint British Societies' risk prediction charts. Similar to most contemporary risk calculators, these charts take account of a range of modifiable and non-modifiable risk factors to estimate the likely risk of an individual developing any type of cardiovascular disease (CVD) (i.e. CHD, stroke or transient cerebral ischaemia) in the next 10 years (Wood et al. 2005). Any patient who has ≥20% risk of developing CVD in the next 10 years should be considered at high risk (Wood et al. 2005).

Once a risk assessment has been carried out, a targeted programme of lifestyle modification and, if necessary, drug therapy can be commenced. One of the benefits of cardiovascular risk charts is that they can demonstrate to individuals the long-term consequences of aspects of their lifestyle, and quantify the benefits of risk factor modification. The NSF for CHD (DH 2000) outlined steps that should be taken for any patient deemed at high risk of cardiac events. All high-risk patients should be given support to modify any factors increasing their risk. Patients who smoke should be offered advice and NRT. Patients should also be educated about the benefits of weight loss, increased physical activity and a healthier diet (DH 2000). All patients at high risk of developing CVD should be offered treatment with statins, with the aim being to maintain an optimum total cholesterol <4.0 mmol/l (Wood et al. 2005, NICE 2006). Drug therapy should also be initiated where necessary to keep BP < 140/85 mmHg (Wood et al. 2005).

SECONDARY PREVENTION

For patients who have had a cardiac event such as an MI, or established heart disease in the form of stable angina, the priority is to try to slow or prevent any further disease progression. As with primary prevention, a major aspect of secondary prevention is support and advice related to lifestyle modification. Pharmacologically, patients will also require a range of different drug therapies. All patients with established CHD should be on low-dose 75 mg aspirin, because this has been shown to reduce the risk of further events significantly (Gaziano et al. 2005). Patients who are allergic or intolerant to aspirin can be prescribed clopidogrel 75 mg daily as an alternative (Dalal et al. 2004). Statins should also be prescribed to reduce total plasma cholesterol by at least 30% (DH 2000). In addition, patients who have had an MI should be prescribed a β blocker, and any patients with left ventricular dysfunction should be treated with an ACE inhibitor (DH 2000). Further details on all these drugs can be found in Chapter 13.

CARDIAC REHABILITATION

Cardiac rehabilitation is a structured process that allows patients with heart disease to achieve their optimum level of health with the support of health professionals (Scottish Intercollegiate Guidelines Network or SIGN 2002). It has been suggested that comprehensive cardiac rehabilitation programmes can reduce cardiac deaths by over 25% (Jolliffe et al. 2001). Given the evidence of clinical effectiveness, patients who have had a cardiac event such as an MI, or who have undergone cardiac surgery, should enter a rehabilitation programme (DH 2000, SIGN 2002). Within the UK, cardiac rehabilitation programmes have traditionally been led within hospitals (Dalal and Evans 2003), recruiting patients after an episode of acute illness or surgery. However, recent developments in cardiac rehabilitation have focused largely on expanding the availability of community- and home-based services. It is this model of seamless cardiac rehabilitation, with services and support available for short-term hospital-based care, before leading into long-term community follow-up, that is widely advocated as the best way forward (De Bono 1998).

In terms of delivery and patient progress, cardiac rehabilitation can be broadly split into four distinct phases.

Phase 1

Phase 1 represents the inpatient stage of the patient journey. This phase will occur in response to a defined change in the patient's usual condition, such as an acute MI or cardiac surgery. During phase 1, a full evaluation of the patient should take place, including consideration of risk factors and the patient's level of knowledge about his or her condition. Education should be provided to ensure that the patient and his or her family understand the implications of the illness, and the future direction of treatment and rehabilitation. Multidisciplinary education and support should also be provided to allow early steps to be taken in the modification of risk factors. Given that phase 1 occurs while the patient is still in hospital, discharge planning is also an element of the care provided (SIGN 2002).

Account should be taken of the patient's psychosocial state. Depression and a feeling of isolation are understandably common after a cardiac event, and their presence can adversely affect recovery rates (Ades 2001). Assessment of psychosocial factors should initially take place during phase 1 of the rehabilitative processes, through either interviews or the use of a formal assessment tool. One of the most common tools used during phase 1 is the Hospital Anxiety and Depression Scale (HADS) – a 14-item questionnaire that gives an indication of a patient's psychological state (SIGN 2002). Screening for psychological symptoms should ideally take place before discharge from hospital, but also at a period 6–12 weeks after the cardiac event, to allow for assessment of patient progress and evaluation of the need for intervention (SIGN 2002). A number of different interventions are used to support patients and their families psychologically after a cardiac event – notably clinical psychologist input, stress management classes and antidepressants (Ades 2001, Dalal et al. 2004).

During phase 1, patients should be educated about the practical changes to their lifestyle that may need to be made. Issues about employment should be addressed, with return to work largely governed by the type of activities inherent in the job (e.g. physical demands, driving). Patients should be made aware of Driving and Vehicle Licensing Agency (DVLA) guidelines on resuming driving after a cardiac event. This varies depending on the condition or type of surgery, and the category of driving licence held. Full details can be found at the DVLA website (www.dvla.gov.uk). Many patients may also have concerns about sexual function after a coronary event. Broadly speaking, patients should wait for about 2 weeks after a cardiac event before assessing their own capability. If they are able to complete an activity such as climbing two flights of stairs without chest pain or breathlessness, then they should be capable of safely having sexual intercourse (McIntosh 2004).

Phase 2

Phase 2 of the cardiac rehabilitation programme relates to the 4- to 6-week period immediately after discharge from hospital (Stokes et al. 1995). All patients should be followed up by telephone, or ideally by a home visit from a specialist cardiac rehabilitation nurse (McIntosh 2004). Patients will often require a significant degree of family and healthcare professional support during phase 2. Discharge from hospital may cause anxiety and stress as the patient is removed from an environment perceived as 'safe'. Patients should receive education about the management and reporting of any cardiac symptoms, and concordance with the exercise and medication regime can also be encouraged. In some areas, patients entering a cardiac rehabilitation programme after an MI utilise a 6-week structured programme known as the 'Heart Manual'. The 'Heart Manual' contains written and audio information for patients and a workbook to track progress. Now widely used in practice, use of the 'Heart Manual' is thought to reduce anxiety and readmission rates after an MI (Lewin 1998).

Phase 3

Phase 3 relates to the intermediate time period after discharge from hospital, and is characterised by a strong emphasis on a structured exercise component. Given the relatively short time period after discharge, most phase 3 exercise programmes have traditionally been run within hospitals, although some areas may provide these services within the community (SIGN 2002). Before starting an exercise programme, patients must be risk stratified. A risk assessment will include consideration of patients' clinical history and current level of symptoms. Investigations such as walking tests, exercise tests or echocardiography may also be used.

The structure of phase 3 programmes will vary between centres, but generally last from 4 to 12 weeks, with one to three exercise sessions per week (McIntosh 2004). The intensity of exercise will vary depending on the individual patient need. Younger patients, or those who wish to carry out physically demanding activity after recovery (e.g. sports), may require a higher-intensity programme. Conversely, patients identified as being at high risk of further cardiac events will usually be suitable only for more moderate intensity exercise. It should also be recognised that some patients may be unsuitable for any form of exercise programme as a result of cardiac instability or poor general clinical condition (SIGN 2002). Although phase 3 of cardiac rehabilitation is often associated largely with an exercise programme, continued multidisciplinary monitoring and support of the patient's psychosocial state and risk status are also necessary.

Phase 4

Phase 4 of the rehabilitative process underpins the long-term progress made by the patient in relation to lifestyle modification and exercise levels. Phase 4 rehabilitation processes are usually managed by primary care practitioners, after formal handover by hospital-based rehabilitation staff (McIntosh 2004). Within phase 4, the support offered to the patient becomes an amalgam of cardiac rehabilitation and secondary prevention, with the dual goals of returning to optimum health while preventing disease progression. Exercise remains an important component of cardiac rehabilitation during phase 4. However, long-term exercise programmes are organised and delivered within community settings such as leisure centres. Long-term monitoring of lifestyle modifications and additional supportive interventions can be delivered by primary care practitioners. Patients in phase 4 also often utilise self-help and support groups, and this should be encouraged (SIGN, 2002).

CONCLUSION

Although much of this book deals with the treatment of cardiac disorders, national policy continues to place greater emphasis on disease prevention. Within the general population, steps are being taken to encourage lower rates of smoking, improve dietary intake and raise levels of physical activity. Patients identified as being at risk of developing CHD must be offered lifestyle advice, accompanied by pharmacological therapy where appropriate. Finally, patients who have already suffered from the effects of CHD must be helped to adjust to the changes in their lifestyle, and given the assistance that they need to readuce to future impact of the disease.

REFERENCES

Ades P (2001) Cardiac rehabilitation and secondary prevention of coronary heart disease. *New England Journal of Medicine* **345**: 892–902.

American Heart Association (1997) Guide to primary prevention of cardiovascular diseases. *Circulation* **95**: 2329–31.

British Heart Foundation (2005) *Coronary Heart Disease Statistics*. Available from www.heartstats.org.

British Obesity Surgery Patient Association (2005) *Weight loss surgery doubles in 2005 but still woefully inadequate say leading patient charity* (press release). Available from www.bospa.org.

Dalal H, Evans P (2003) Achieving national service framework standards for cardiac rehabilitation and secondary prevention. *British Medical Journal* **326**: 481–4.

Dalal H, Evans P, Campbell J (2004) Recent developments in secondary prevention and cardiac rehabilitation after acute myocardial infarction. *British Medical Journal* **328**: 693–7.

De Bono D (1998) Models of cardiac rehabilitation. Multidisciplinary rehabilitation is worthwhile, but how is it best delivered? *British Medical Journal* **316**: 1329–30.

Department of Health (2000) *National Service Framework for Coronary Heart Disease.* London: Department of Health.

Department of Health (2004) *At Least Five a Week: Evidence on the impact of physical activity and its relationship to health.* London: Department of Health.

European Society of Cardiology (2003) European guidelines on cardiovascular disease prevention in clinical practice. *European Heart Journal* **24**: 1601–10.

Gaw A, Shepherd J (2004) Lipids and lipid lowering drugs. In: Lindsay G, Gaw A (eds), *Coronary Heart Disease Prevention*, 2nd edn. Edinburgh: Churchill Livingstone, pp 53–73.

Gaziano J, Manson J, Ridker P (2005) Primary and secondary prevention of coronary heart disease. In: Zipes D, Libby P, Bonow R, Braunwald E (eds), *Braunwald's Heart Disease*, 7th edn. Philadelphia: WB Saunders, pp 1057–84.

Gibson M (2003) Managing CHD risk in people with diabetes. *Cardiology News* **6**(3): 10–13.

Gordon MB, Libby P (2003) Atherosclerosis. In: Lilly L (ed.), *Pathophysiology of Heart Disease*, 3rd edn. Philadelphia: Lippincott, Williams & Wilkins, pp 111–30.

Griffin B, Whitehead K (2004) Lifestyle management: diet. In: Lindsay G, Gaw A (eds), *Coronary Heart Disease Prevention*, 2nd edn. Edinburgh: Churchill Livingstone, pp 159–87.

Grønbaek M (2004) Wine, alcohol and cardiovascular risk: open issue. *Journal of Thrombosis and Haemostasis* **2**: 2041–2.

Hatchett R, Thompson D (eds) (2002) The sociological and human impact of coronary heart disease. In: *Cardiac Nursing: A comprehensive guide*. Edinburgh: Churchill Livingstone, pp 3–13.

Health Development Agency (2001) *Coronary Heart Disease. Guidance for implementing the preventative aspects of the National Service Framework.* London: HDA.

Hobbs F (2004) Cardiovascular disease: Different strategies for primary and secondary prevention? *Heart* **90**: 1217–23.

Jolliffe J, Rees K, Taylor D, Oldridge N, Ebrahim S (2001) Exercise-based rehabilitation for coronary heart disease. *Cochrane Database of Systematic Reviews* Issue 1.

Lewin B (1998) *Cardiac Rehabilitation, A Cognitive Behavioural Model, the Heart Manual and Other Topics.* Available from www.cardiacrehabilitation.org.uk/heart_manual/chapter.htm.

Lindsay G (2004) Risk factor assessment. In: Lindsay G, Gaw A (eds), *Coronary Heart Disease Prevention*, 2nd edn. Edinburgh: Churchill Livingstone, pp 29–52.

McIntosh L (2004) Cardiac rehabilitation. In: Lindsay G, Gaw A (eds), *Coronary Heart Disease Prevention*, 2nd edn. Edinburgh: Churchill Livingstone, pp 271–86.

Maron D, Grundy S, Ridker P, Pearson T (2004) Dyslipidemia, other risk factors, and the prevention of coronary heart disease. In: Fuster V, Wayne Alexander R, O'Rourke R (eds), *Hurst's The Heart*, 11th edn. New York: McGraw-Hill, pp 1093–122.

National Institute for Clinical Excellence (2001a) *Guidance on the Use of Orlistat for the Treatment of Obesity in Adults*. London: NICE.

National Institute for Clinical Excellence (2001b) *Guidance on the Use of Sibutramine for the Treatment of Obesity in Adults*. London: NICE.

National Institute for Clinical Excellence (2002a) *Guidance on the Use of Nicotine Replacement Therapy (NRT) and Bupropion in Smoking Cessation*. London: NICE.

National Institute for Clinical Excellence (2002b) *Guidance on the Use of Surgery to Aid Weight Reduction for People with Morbid Obesity*. London: NICE.

National Institute for Health and Clinical Excellence (2006) *Statins for the Prevention of Cardiovascular Events.* London: NICE.

SIGN (2002) *Cardiac Rehabilitation: A national clinical guideline*. Edinburgh: SIGN.

Stokes H, Turner S, Farr A (1995) Cardiac rehabilitation: programme structure, content, management and administration. In: Coats A, McGee H, Stokes H, Thompson D (eds), *British Association for Cardiac Rehabilitation Guidelines for Cardiac Rehabilitation* Oxford: Blackwell Science, pp 12–39.

Thompson G (2004) Management of dyslipidaemia. *Heart* **90**: 949–55.

Thompson D, Webster R (2004) *Caring for the Coronary Patient*, 2nd edn. Edinburgh: Butterworth Heinemann.

Williams B, Poulter N, Brown M et al. (2004) British Hypertension Society guidelines for hypertension management 2004 (BHS IV): summary. *British Medical Journal* **328**: 634–40.

Wood D, Wray R, Poulter N et al. (2005) JBS 2: Joint British Societies' guidelines on prevention of cardiovascular disease in clinical practice. *Heart* **91**(suppl V): v1–52.

World Health Organization (2004) *The Atlas of Heart Disease and Stroke.* Geneva: WHO.

4 Anatomy and physiology of the heart

MARK GRETTON

Throughout recorded history the heart has been viewed by scientists, poets and lovers as at the centre of all things physical and emotional, and sometimes as even transcending man. The bible records God being pleased 'in his heart' by Noah's sacrifice after the safe delivery of the ark from the flood, and resolving to make a covenant with man 'even though every inclination of his [man's] heart is evil from childhood' (*The Holy Bible* 1978a, p 8). In the New Testament, the apostle Paul encourages members of the new church at Ephesus to 'Sing and make music in your heart to the Lord' (*The Holy Bible* 1978b, p 1199). The ancient Egyptians believed that Ptah, the chief god of the ancient city of Memphis, brought all things into being by conceiving of them in his heart and speaking them into existence. More prosaically, they believed that the heart 'spoke in the vessel of all the [body's] members' (McDevitt 2006), which may indicate an understanding of the relationship between the heart and the pulse. Not surprisingly, they felt that the heart held the mind and soul of an individual. During mummification rituals, although almost all organs, including the brain, were removed, the heart was always left in the body (McDevitt 2006). More recently, the idea of the heart as the centre of the person has been revived in the intriguing cases of heart transplant recipients who seem to gain memories of the life of the heart donor (Pearsall et al. 2000). Romantically, the heart is seen as a metaphor for love as heart strings are tugged and, from Shakespeare to The Smiths (*Asleep*, from the album *The Smiths: Louder than bombs*), a broken heart is synonymous with love unrequited or betrayed (Craig 1905).

Rather more prosaically, the heart can usefully be compared with a central heating system (albeit an unusually efficient one), a pump propelling fluid round a system of pipes and regulated by an electric timer. Regardless of how far we subscribe to far-reaching, mystical or romantic notions, the heart is a remarkable piece of human machinery, ensuring through its contractions a sufficient supply of oxygenated blood to the rest of the body to allow all the other organs to function. Over the lifetime of a person living to 75 years of age, and

Cardiac Care: An Introduction for Healthcare Professionals. Edited by David Barrett, Mark Gretton and Tom Quinn
© 2006 John Wiley & Sons Ltd

having an average heart rate of 70 beats per minute, this requires the heart to beat more than 2.7 billion times.

In this chapter I examine the structure and function of the heart at both systemic and cellular levels, and consider the complex interplay of the mechanical and the electrical systems of the heart.

THE GENERAL ANATOMY OF THE HEART

The heart is a hollow, cone-shaped, fibromuscular organ about the size of an adult fist and weighing around 340 g (Thompson and Webster 2004). It is positioned in the middle mediastinal compartment of the thorax between the two pleural cavities, which almost completely overlap it. Two-thirds of it is positioned to the left of the midline of the body, and the long axis of the heart is positioned downwards, leftwards, obliquely and forwards (Bond 2000). Anything that changes the shape of the chest, be it positioning, disease or weight changes, will alter the position and shape of the heart. Often tall, thin people have a more vertical heart than short, fat people (Bond 2000). The heart is encased by the pericardium, a fibroserous sac. The tough, outer layer of the pericardium – the fibrous pericardium – is anchored to the sternum and the pleura, helping to hold the heart in its place. Inside this is a double-layered sac, the serous pericardium, which is composed of a parietal and a visceral layer. The parietal pericardium tightly adheres to the inner surface of the fibrous pericardium, whereas the visceral pericardium makes up the outer surface of the heart and is also sometimes referred to as the epicardium. This consists of a single layer of mesothelial cells supported by a thin layer of connective tissue with elastic fibres, blood vessels and nerve ganglia (Guyton 1991). The potential distance between the parietal and visceral layers is called the pericardial space and contains a thin film of 10–50 ml serous fluid, which serves as a lubricant, preventing the heart from being damaged by its own contractions (Price and Wilson 1992).

Inside the pericardium is the myocardium, a thick, muscular layer interspersed with connective tissue and small blood vessels. The myocardium is both the nerve centre and the powerhouse of cardiac tissue, responsible for both the generation and the conduction of cardiac impulses, and for cardiac contraction. The innermost layer is the endocardium, a single layer of endothelial cells interspersed with a few layers of collagen and elastic fibres that form the surface of the heart valves and the interior of the heart chambers (Figure 4.1).

THE FOUR CHAMBERS OF THE HEART

There are four chambers in the heart, the right and left atria and the right and left ventricles. After the changes of birth there is no direct communication

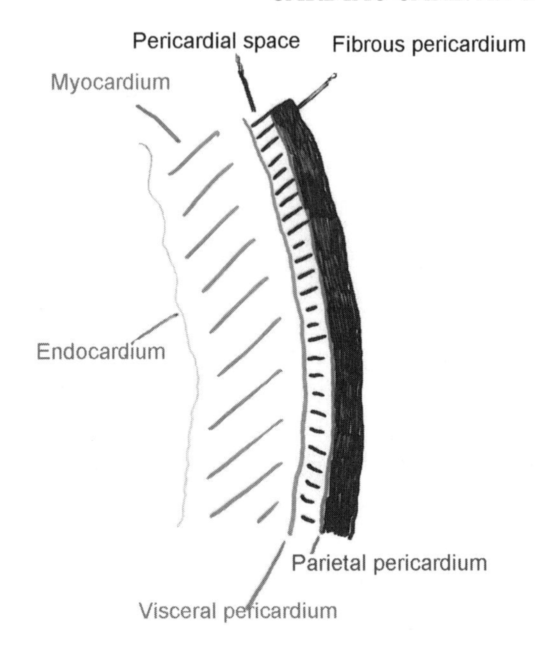

Figure 4.1 Layers of the heart.

between the right and left heart, the ventricles being separated by the muscular interventricular septum. Blood moves from the right atrium to the right ventricle and from the left atrium to the left ventricle. The right ventricle moves blood to the lungs and the left ventricle moves blood round the body. Given that the distance that it has to move the blood and the pressures against which it has to move it are much greater than those of the other chambers, the wall of the left ventricle is much thicker than that of the other chambers, typically 13–15 mm, compared with 2 mm for the right atrium, 3 mm for the left atrium and 3–5 mm for the right ventricle.

THE HEART VALVES

For blood to move through the heart efficiently, there is a system of valves to prevent blood leaking backwards. The tricuspid valve has three leaflets and prevents blood from being propelled from the right ventricle back into the right atrium. The pulmonary valve is sometimes called a semi-lunar valve, because its two leaflets are half-moon shaped and it stops blood flowing back from the pulmonary artery into the right ventricle. The bicuspid (two leaflets) valve that stops blood being propelled back from the left ventricle into the left atrium is most commonly called the mitral valve, because it has been said to resemble a bishop's hat, or mitre. The tricuspid and mitral valves are referred to as atrioventricular valves, and both are anchored to the endocardial wall of the heart by fibrous cords called chordae tendineae; these are string-like in appearance and are the 'heart strings' mentioned earlier, attaching these valves to the papillary muscles and ventricular walls (Cardiovascular Consultants 2006). The aortic valve prevents blood from leaking back from the aorta to the left ventricle and is another semi-lunar valve. If you find, as many do, difficulty at first in remembering the sequence of the valves related to blood flow, you might find a mnemonic based on the initial letters useful (**t**ricuspid, **p**ulmonary, **m**itral, **a**ortic), such as The Poor Man's Arm (or similar).

THE FLOW OF BLOOD THROUGH THE HEART

Blood drains into the heart from the systemic circulation via the superior and inferior venae cavae. The superior vena cava brings deoxygenated blood from the head, neck, arm and chest regions of the body to the right atrium; the inferior vena cava does the same from the lower regions of the body. They drain, respectively, into the upper and lower parts of the right atrium and pass through the tricuspid valve into the right ventricle. The right ventricle then ejects blood via the pulmonary valve into the pulmonary artery and to the lungs. The pulmonary artery is thus the only artery of the body to purvey deoxygenated blood. The blood is then oxygenated by the lungs and drained back to the left atrium via four pulmonary veins, two from each lung. The pulmonary veins are therefore also unusual in that they carry oxygenated rather than deoxygenated blood, as other veins do. In the light of this, it is useful to think of arteries as taking blood away from the heart and veins bringing blood to the heart (Cardiovascular Consultants 2006).

From the left atrium blood moves through to the left ventricle via the mitral valve; the left ventricle then ejects it through the aortic valve and into the aorta, from whence it proceeds to oxygenate the organs and tissues of the body.

THE CORONARY CIRCULATION

The first organ supplied with oxygenated blood is the heart itself. The heart uses a tremendous amount of energy to function as a pump; this energy is garnered from adenosine triphosphate (ATP) and produced by oxidative metabolism. Thus, the heart requires a large and continuous supply of oxygen and soon becomes distressed if this supply is interrupted, being unable to sustain an oxygen debt in the way that skeletal muscle can (Thompson and Webster 2004). Two coronary arteries branch directly from the aorta – the right coronary artery (RCA) and the left coronary artery (LCA). However, functionally and for convenience, the bifurcation of the LCA into the left anterior descending (LAD) branch and the circumflex (Cx) branch means that often clinicians will refer to three coronary arteries.

The right and left coronary arteries supply the heart with around 4% of the output of the left ventricle during diastole. As with so much about the heart, this is perhaps not the full picture, because some studies have indicated a direct communication between the chambers of the heart and the coronary arteries, opening up the intriguing possibility that the heart nourishes itself in part from blood in the ventricles draining via myocardial sinusoids directly into the coronary arteries (Wearn et al. 1933), although there is contradictory evidence to this (Smith 1962).

In general, the RCA supplies the right atrium and ventricle and the LCA the left atrium and ventricle. The RCA also normally supplies most of the conduction system of the heart, usually around 55% of the sinoatrial (SA) node and 90% of the atrioventricular (AV) node and the bundle of His (Bond 2000). This is why early bradyarrhythmic complications after a heart attack are more common in inferior or posterior myocardial infarction than in anterior infarction, because the inferior and posterior walls of the heart are normally predominantly supplied by the RCA whereas the anterior wall is usually mainly supplied by the LCA (Rosenfeld 1988). Despite this, overall prognosis is worse in the longer term for anterior infarctions, probably as a result of involving the larger muscular mass of the left ventricle (Haim et al. 1997).

Although the LCA generally supplies the largest muscular mass and has a wider bore than the RCA, the RCA is generally described as dominant. This is because dominance, in this circumstance, is an anatomical rather than a physiological term and refers to whichever of the coronary arteries reaches beyond the crux, the area of the back of the heart where the right and left AV grooves cross the interatrial and interventricular grooves. In around 85–90% of people this is the RCA, regardless of whether or not it is supplying the most blood (Nerantzis et al. 1996).

THE CONDUCTION SYSTEM OF THE HEART

The heart is often described as a muscular pump, but although this is a useful description it is also a considerable over-simplification. First, the heart is in effect two muscular pumps, interconnected but separate, the right propelling blood to the lungs and the left sending blood round the body. Second, the pumping activity of both sides is regulated by an electrical activity that, although it does not power the pumps, can be said to initiate the pumping action, acting as the heart's pacemaker. This electrical activity can be regarded as another system within the heart, containing its own structures made up of cells that are significantly different from other cardiac cells.

The principal pacemaker area of the heart is normally the SA node, named from its position at the junction of the superior vena cava and the right atrium. The SA node initiates impulses that spread across the heart. As they spread, they reach other conduction cells and cause them to depolarise and, when they reach myocardial cells, they cause them to contract, producing muscular activity. The pacemaker cells do not have a real contractile element and as such they do not themselves contribute significantly to cardiac contraction. The impulses from the SA node spread across the atria and are then 'picked up' at the AV node, situated at the junction of the atria and the ventricles. The AV node is particularly important in that it slows down conduction through the heart, acting as a brake on the wave of depolarisation spreading across the heart. This means, in normal conduction, that ventricular excitation does not take place until the atria have had time to contract. It also means that, in the case of abnormally rapid heart rhythms initiated above the AV node, a limited number of these impulses are transmitted through to the ventricles. Thus tachycardias initiated above the ventricles (e.g. narrow complex or supraventricular tachycardias), although they may be uncomfortably fast for the sufferer, are not usually dangerously fast (see Chapter 9 for more details about tachycardias).

Impulses from the AV node then pass into the AV bundle, which is sometimes called the bundle of His. This stretches down the interventricular septum and separates into the left and right bundle branches, which carry impulses across the ventricles. The left bundle branch itself quickly bifurcates into an anterior and posterior branch, whereas the right bundle branch remains common for longer. The right and left bundle branches carry impulses respectively across the right and left ventricles, finally breaking down into a system of microscopic fibres that convey the impulses, often referred to as Purkinje fibres.

CARDIAC CELLS

The specialist cells that make up the pacemaker system described above have the capacity to initiate an electrical impulse, the quality of automaticity. All cardiac cells can transmit or conduct impulses, but the pacemaker cells are able to do this in a more rapid and more coordinated way than the other cells. Thus, impulses are initiated by the pacemaker cells and conducted by other pacemaker cells to prompt contraction in contractile myocardial cells. All cardiac cells have to conduct impulses, so that the impulses can spread completely across the heart. This happens because cardiac cells are so closely packed together that an impulse initiated in one will immediately affect the next and then the next, so that the electrical impulse spreads like a wave.

These electrical changes are caused by ionic changes in the cells. The cells are either positively or negatively charged and the concentrations of the different ions affect the charge both inside and outside a cell (Levick 2000). To cause an electrical impulse to move from one cell to another, and to cause contraction in contractile cells (sometimes called worker cells), these ionic changes have to be dramatic enough to trigger an action potential.

ACTION POTENTIAL IN MYOCARDIAL 'WORKER' CELLS

The ions principally involved in evoking an action potential in myocardial worker cells are sodium (Na^+), potassium (K^+) and calcium (Ca^{2+}), all of which carry a positive charge. Other ions, such as the negatively charged chloride (Cl^-), have a lesser role. When a cell is at rest, i.e. polarised, the charge in it is negative, around –90 mV. For a cell to depolarise it undergoes a number of distinct ionic changes that alter the charge within the cell.

Phase 4: polarisation (Figure 4.2)

This is the resting or recovery phase and so we can consider it to be the first phase before the intracellular changes that cause the action potential. The polarisation is actively maintained by the Na^+/K^+ pump, fuelled by ATP, whereby Na^+ is pumped in and K^+ is pumped out. Therefore the cell's electrical charge is kept at around –90 mV. Although the intracellular space is relatively negative, the extracellular space is relatively positive.

Phase 0: depolarisation (Figure 4.3)

Membrane permeability to sodium is markedly increased at this point, allowing positively charged sodium ions to rush in, so that the cellular charge changes from –90 mV to –60 mV. This is referred to as the threshold potential, the point of no return for the cell, because membrane permeability is further increased to allow a secondary influx of Na^+ ions along with an influx of Ca^{2+} ions. The cell is now positively charged at around +20 to +30 mV, whereas the

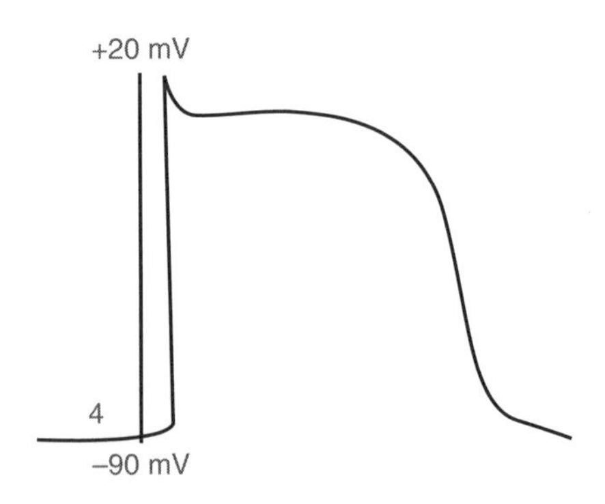

Figure 4.2 Phase 4: polarisation.

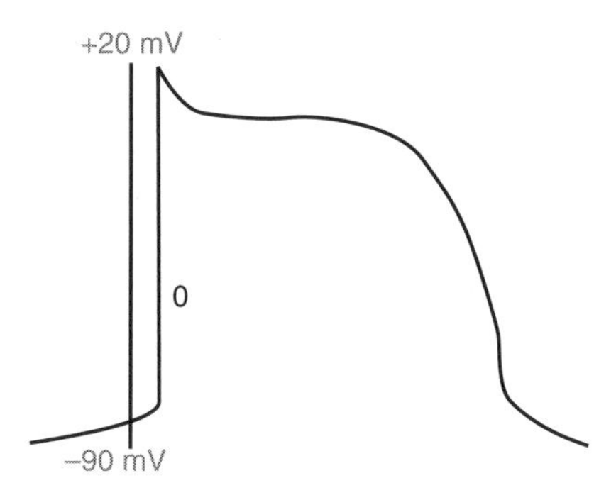

Figure 4.3 Phase 0: depolarisation.

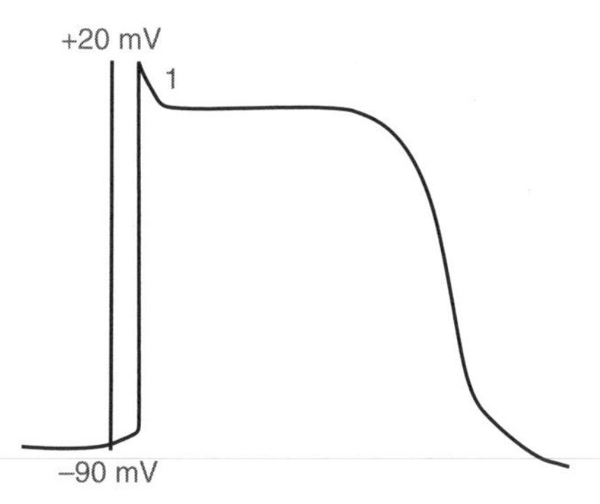

Figure 4.4 Phase 1: overshoot.

extracellular space is negatively charged. This is a reverse of the surrounding cells, so a potential difference exists, allowing current to flow to the next cell.

Phase 1: overshoot (Figure 4.4)

Phase 1 is the first of three phases of repolarisation. Negatively charged Cl^- ions enter the cells at this point, causing the electrical potential to fall to around +10 mV. At this stage the fast Na^+ channels have become inactive, so there is no further rapid influx of Na^+.

Phase 2: plateau (Figure 4.5)

The membrane remains depolarised at this stage. This is the absolute refractory period, the time during which cells cannot normally depolarise. There is a slow influx of Ca^{2+} and an influx of Na^+ through slow channels, but the balance is maintained by K^+ moving outwards.

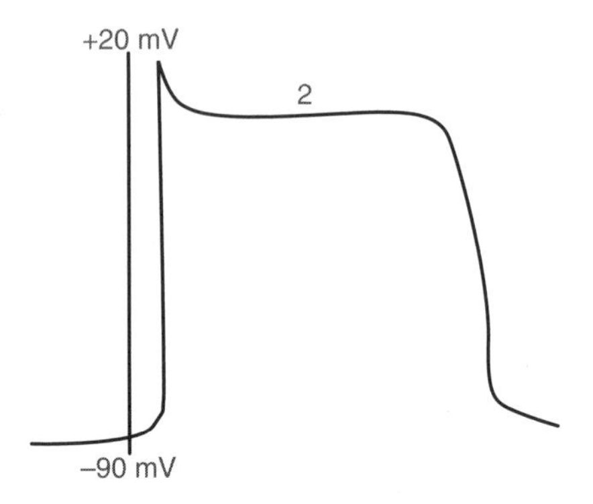

Figure 4.5 Phase 2: plateau.

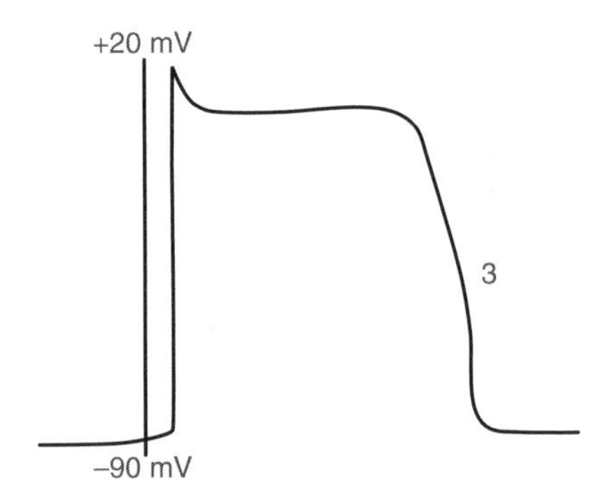

Figure 4.6 Phase 3: rapid potassium efflux.

Phase 3: rapid potassium efflux (Figure 4.6)

The slow inward current of Ca^{2+} and Na^{+} finishes and K^{+} leaves the cell much more rapidly, thus reducing the positive charge within it. The membrane potential rapidly returns to –90 mV and the action potential is ended.

Depolarisation in pacemaker cells (Figure 4.7)

As mentioned earlier, these cells can initiate a spontaneous electrical response. As a result of this, phase 4 does not properly exist in pacemaker cells. Instead there is an unstable resting phase with slow, spontaneous depolarisation, caused by a slow, continuous movement of Na^{+} into these cells during diastole, until the threshold potential is reached.

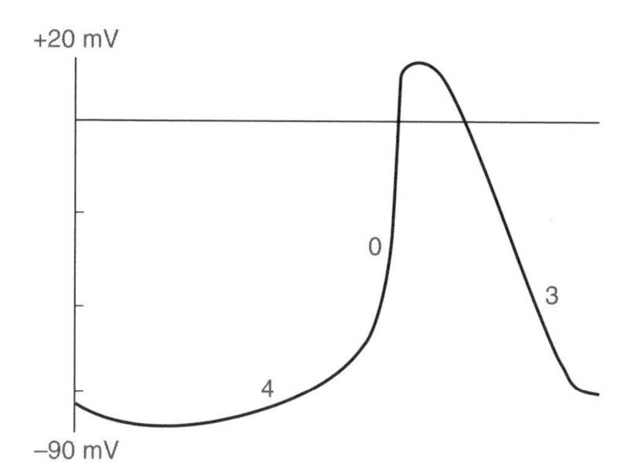

Figure 4.7 Depolarisation in pacemaker cells.

Excitation–contraction coupling

Electrical excitation, the evoking of an action potential described above, leads to cardiac muscle contraction. The linkage between electrical activity and cardiac contraction is complicated and based on a number of factors, and is referred to as excitation–contraction coupling.

Cardiac cells are composed of fine fibres called myofibrils. These consist of small contractile units called sarcomeres. The sarcomeres consist of two contractile proteins, actin and myosin. Myosin is a thick filament that overlaps a thin filament consisting of actin and two regulatory proteins, tropomyosin and troponin. The myosin filaments contain cross-bridges that 'jut out' towards the actin filaments and binding sites. When cardiac muscle is relaxed, the tropomyosin/troponin complex covers the actin-binding sites, so the myosin cross-bridges are unable to bind to the actin (Guyton 1991); no cross-bridges therefore means that there is no contraction.

Contraction is activated by Ca^{2+} stored in the longitudinal tubules of the cardiac cells. Troponin and Ca^{2+} have a strong affinity, so they bind together and uncover the actin-binding sites, allowing the myosin cross-bridges to link up with the actin. These bridges break and re-form, each time drawing the layers of actin closer together, thus causing cardiac muscle contraction by what has been called the 'sliding filament' mechanism (Levick 2000) (Figure 4.8).

An appreciation of these mechanisms helps in understanding some important properties of cardiac tissue and cardiac activity. What is often referred to as the Frank–Starling law (Thompson and Webster 2004) states that cardiac muscle fibres contract more forcibly the more they are stretched before the start of contraction, within physiological limits. This is because, as actin and myosin fibres are pulled further apart, more actin-binding sites are revealed and able to participate in the process of contraction. Unfortunately, beyond a

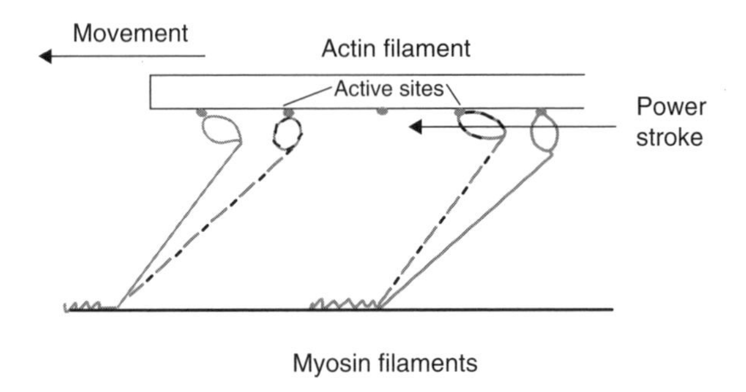

Figure 4.8 The 'sliding filament' mechanism for contraction of cardiac muscle.

certain point the filaments will become so over-stretched that fewer and fewer binding sites link the filaments together, so contraction becomes weaker.

A useful analogy is with elasticated underwear. Normally it fits snugly and, if stretched further, will recoil with a satisfying snap. But if it is repeatedly stretched beyond a certain point, it eventually loses its power of recoil and becomes loose and baggy; ultimately it is not to be relied upon to stay in place and do the job required of it. Similarly the heart will initially respond to a greater volume of blood (preload) and a greater pressure to be overcome in ejecting the blood (afterload) by stretching its fibres and contracting with more vigour (increasing contractility) and so the stroke volume (SV), the amount of blood the left ventricle ejects each beat, will increase. This is not sustainable indefinitely and eventually the heart will fail and contract with less force and cardiac output (CO) will decrease.

Preload is the load or volume of blood in the ventricles at the end of diastole and is sometimes referred to as left-ventricular end-diastolic pressure (LVEDP) or left ventricular filling pressure (LVFP). Afterload is the resistance against which the ventricle has to pump and is related to factors such as aortic impedance, peripheral vascular resistance and blood viscosity.

The role of Ca^{2+} in both action potential changes and contraction is clearly vital and it would appear to have a further role in what is sometimes called the 'Treppe' or 'staircase' phenomenon (Wussling and Syzmanski 1986). Tissue experiments have shown that, if the cardiac preload is kept constant, contractility increases as heart rate (HR) increases (Figure 4.9). Generally speaking, an increase in HR will cause an increase in CO, but beyond a certain rate the time that the left ventricle has to fill will shorten to a point where CO may fall as a result of there being less blood to eject. The Treppe phenomenon may protect the heart from this by ensuring that as much as possible of the blood filling the heart is ejected by the increased contractile power of the ventricle. This may be caused by rate-regulated increases in Ca^{2+} uncovering extra, active binding sites.

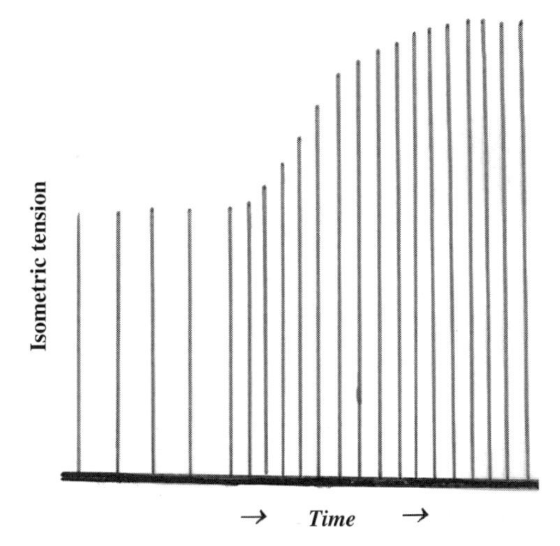

Figure 4.9 The 'ascending staircase' of the Treppe phenomenon, as increased heart rate (i.e. shorter time between impulses) causes increased contraction (i.e. isometric tension).

Cardiac output

Putting the above together, we can see that CO can be calculated using the formula:

$$CO = HR \times SV.$$

Thus in a normal adult at rest, a heart rate of 70 beats/min (bpm) combined with an SV of 80 ml blood per contraction would produce a CO of 5.6 l/min. Increases in HR and contraction caused by exercise, stress or disease will greatly increase or decrease CO, as will changes to SV caused by such factors as valvular disease, peripheral circulation and blood viscosity.

PUTTING IT ALL TOGETHER – THE CARDIAC CYCLE

The cardiac cycle refers to the sequential activation of the cardiac chambers through the coordinated functioning of the electrical and muscular changes described. Broadly speaking, the cycle is divided into ventricular systole (when the ventricle contracts) and ventricular diastole (when it does not) but it is helpful to consider the different phases of these events. For simplicity's sake I consider in detail only the left ventricular cardiac cycle, because, although the sequence of events is the same in both ventricles, the timings are slightly different as a result of factors such as the different pressures within the respective ventricles (Bond 2000). Given that this is a continuous cycle I could start a description of it anywhere, but for convention's sake I begin with ventricular systole.

VENTRICULAR SYSTOLE

Isovolumic ventricular contraction (0.05 seconds)

This follows ventricular depolarisation as represented by the start of the QRS complex on the ECG. Ventricular pressure increases rapidly, while the atrial pressure decreases with atrial relaxation and repolarisation. The mitral valve closes and pressure in the ventricle becomes higher than in the atrium. The aortic valve is closed. The ventricle increases in size but the blood volume is not altered, because there is no flow in or out.

Rapid ventricular ejection (0.09 seconds)

The contraction of the ventricular muscle continues and the aortic valve opens when ventricular pressure exceeds aortic pressure (about 80 mmHg). The ventricle and the aorta are common cavities at this stage. Ventricular pressure rises to 120 mmHg and two-thirds of the SV is ejected during this period. Aortic pressure may exceed ventricular pressure at the end of this period, but blood flow continues through forward momentum. Most of the SV is accommodated in the elastic proximal aorta. The atrium is relaxed, but the pressure begins to rise as blood from the lungs accumulates and ventricular repolarisation begins.

Reduced ventricular ejection (0.13 seconds)

Ventricular and aortic pressures decrease as ventricular fibres no longer contract as forcefully as they have done because they have reached a shorter length. Ventricular volume continues to fall, but the blood flow to the aorta carries on, although at a slower rate. Ventricular repolarisation is completed by this time, as indicated by the end of the T wave on the ECG.

VENTRICULAR DIASTOLE

Protodiastole (0.04 seconds)

Ventricular muscle relaxation begins, so ventricular pressure falls below aortic pressure. Blood therefore tries to flow back into the ventricle, which causes the aortic valve to shut. There is a slight transient decrease in atrial pressure, reflecting ventricular relaxation.

Isovolumic ventricular relaxation (0.08 seconds)

Ventricular pressure now decreases rapidly as the ventricle relaxes. There is no change in ventricular volume because all valves are closed. After closure of the aortic valve, aortic pressure rises (causing a dicrotic notch on a pressure tracing) and atrial pressure continues to rise as the atrium receives blood from the lungs.

Rapid ventricular filling (0.11 seconds)

The mitral valve opens when ventricular pressure drops below atrial pressure. The ventricle fills rapidly with blood, but the ventricular pressure continues to fall, as ventricular relaxation continues. Most of the atrial blood has emptied into the ventricle by the time the ventricle reaches its maximum diastolic size. Atrial pressure decreases as the atrium empties, but remains slightly higher than ventricular pressure.

Late diastole (diastasis) (0.19 seconds)

The mitral valve remains open and the pressures within the atrium and the ventricle equilibrate at this time. Blood from the lungs continues to enter the ventricle passively and ventricular volume and pressure gradually rise. Coronary artery blood flow is maximal at this time, which is the beginning of atrial depolarisation, as signalled by the upstroke of the P wave on the ECG.

Atrial contraction (0.11 seconds)

After ventricular diastole, the atrial muscle contracts, increasing atrial pressure. Although most of the ventricular filling has been accomplished by changes to the pressure gradient, a further 15–25% of blood is ejected from the atrium at this point. Aortic pressure continues to decrease as blood flows from it to the peripheries. As this ends, the ventricle starts to depolarise again and so the cycle is repeated, over 2.7 billion times in the average lifetime.

CONCLUSION

The heart is a remarkable organ, a complex system of two interlinked but separately functioning pumps regulated electrically. Through a sequential activation of its systems of chambers and valves it moves blood drained from the venous circulation to the lungs to be oxygenated, and then round the body in order to nourish all of the body's cells, tissues and organs.

REFERENCES

Bond E (2000) Cardiac anatomy and physiology. In: Woods SL, Froelicher E, Motzer S (eds), *Cardiac Nursing,* 4th edn. Philadelphia: Lippincott, Williams & Wilkins, pp 3–49.

Cardiovascular Consultants (2006) *Heart anatomy*. Available from www.cardioconsult.com/Anatomy .

Craig WJ (1905) *The Oxford Shakespeare Complete Works*. London: Oxford University Press.

Guyton AC (1991) *Textbook of Medical Physiology*, 8th edn. Philadelphia: WB Saunders.

Haim M, Hod H, Reisin L et al. (1997) Comparison of short- and long-term prognosis in patients with anterior wall versus inferior or lateral wall non-Q-wave acute myocardial infarction. Secondary Prevention Reinfarction Israeli Nifedipine Trial (SPRINT) Study Group. *American Journal of Cardiology* **15**: 717–21.

Levick JR (2000) *An Introduction to Cardiovascular Physiology*. London: Arnold.

McDevitt A (2006) *Ancient Egypt: The mythology (the heart)*. Available from www.egyptianmyths.net/heart.htm.

Nerantzis C, Papachristos J, Gribizi J et al. (1996) Functional dominance of the right coronary artery: incidence in the human heart. *Clinical Anatomy* **9**(1): 10–13.

Pearsall P, Schwartz G, Russek L (2000) Changes in heart transplant recipients that parallel the personalities of their donors. *Integrative Medicine* **21**(2): 65–72.

Price S, Wilson L (eds) (1992) *Pathophysiology*. St Louis, MO: Mosby.

Rosenfeld LE (1988) Bradyarrhythmias, abnormalities of conduction, and indications for pacing in acute myocardial infarction. *Cardiology Clinics* **6**(1): 49–61.

Smith GT (1962) The anatomy of the coronary circulation. *American Journal of Cardiology* **9**: 327–42.

The Holy Bible (1978a) *Genesis* 8:21. New International Version. London: Hodder & Stoughton.

The Holy Bible (1978b) *Ephesians* 5:19. New International Version. London: Hodder & Stoughton.

Thompson D, Webster R (2004) *Caring for the Cardiac Patient*, 2nd edn. Edinburgh: Butterworth-Heinemann.

Wearn J, Mettier S, Klumpp T, Zschiesche L (1933) The nature of the vascular communications between the coronary arteries and the chambers of the heart. *American Heart Journal* **IX**(2): 143–64.

Wussling M, Szymanski G (1986) Simulation by two calcium store models of myocardial dynamic properties: potentiation, staircase, and biphasic tension development. *General Physiology and Biophysics* **5**(2): 135–52.

5 Assessing the cardiac patient

MARK GRETTON

The skills required to assess effectively someone with an actual or suspected cardiac problem are among the most important that those caring for these patients need to develop. Much of the effective management of these patients depends on the ability of those caring for them quickly and accurately to assess their cardiovascular state. Whether practitioners are then in a position to intervene to help the patient, or whether they have to pass the information on to someone else, it is essential that they recognise changes from the normal and understand what they mean.

In this chapter I look at how to assess the clinical signs and symptoms of a deteriorating patient, how to recognise ischaemic pain and differentiate it from other similar pain presentations, and how to use and interpret the ECG. I focus on what such assessment and monitoring tells us about the patient in front of us and what we need to do to help this patient.

ASSESSING THE DETERIORATING PATIENT

Before looking in depth at specific cardiac conditions, we must consider these in the context of the general deterioration of the patient 'at risk'. Over the last few years it has become apparent that health practitioners are not particularly skilled in assessing at-risk patients or, if they do have the appropriate assessment skills, all too often they have not realised the importance of rapid intervention once deterioration has been observed. The failure to recognise what are sometimes called 'early warning signs' (Department of Health or DH 2000) has undoubtedly led to both unnecessary admissions to intensive care units (ICUs) and unnecessary deaths (McQuillen et al. 1998, McArthur-Rouse 2001, Harrison et al. 2005). It is important to be aware of generalised signs of deterioration when assessing a patient because so often causes of deterioration have a cardiovascular origin or, if they have not been caused by a primary cardiac problem, they quickly have a profound and damaging effect on the heart.

There are a number of ways in which a practitioner can quickly and effectively analyse a deteriorating patient. I focus on the 'ABCDE' method, a

Cardiac Care: An Introduction for Healthcare Professionals. Edited by David Barrett, Mark Gretton and Tom Quinn
© 2006 John Wiley & Sons Ltd

variation of which has been taught for some years on resuscitation courses sanctioned by the Resuscitation Council (UK) (2006). The 'ABCDE' (**a**irway, **b**reathing, **c**irculation, **d**isability, **e**xposure) method of assessment requires, in effect, that practitioners ask themselves a number of sequential questions about patients in front of them and, if the answer to any of them is 'yes', to ask if there is anything that they can do to remedy the problems that they have found. Finally, whatever the success of intervention, it requires that they ensure that the appropriate expert help is on the way as soon as possible.

Airway

- Is the airway threatened?
- Is the person silent, does breathing sound extremely noisy, or does it rattle or gurgle?
- Is there blood or vomit around the person's nose or mouth, which might indicate that the airway is blocked by a foreign body such as food?
- Are there obvious signs of injury to the nose, mouth or throat, indicative of trauma to the airway?
- Do the face and throat appear reddened and swollen, which may be evidence of infection or inflammation to the airway?

If any of the above signs are present you must try to remedy them immediately by attempting to protect the airway (Jaworski 2002).

- Can the mouth be opened safely? If so, can you see any foreign body blocking the airway that can be moved either by a finger sweep or the use of aids such as long forceps, or by chest compressions if the patient has lost consciousness?
- If the airway is compromised by fluids, can these be suctioned away?
- If this is not possible, can the casualty be safely turned on to the side, so that fluids can drain safely out of the nose and mouth?
- Can the airway be opened by performing the head-tilt, chin-lift manoeuvre or by using a jaw thrust?
- Once the airway has been opened, can it be made safer by siting an adjunct such as an oropharyngeal or nasopharyngeal airway, or a laryngeal mask airway (Bein and Scholtz 2005)?

Breathing

- Is the patient breathing at all when you perform a 10-second check by looking to see if the chest is rising or falling, listening for sounds of breathing and feeling whether there is breath on your hand or face? If the patient is not breathing, help must be called and basic life support commenced as described in Chapter 10.
- If the patient is breathing, is the rate much slower or faster than it was when you last checked (Smith and Wood 1998)?

- If you do not know this, is the patient extremely tachypnoeic, with a rate of 40 breaths/minute or more, or profoundly bradypnoeic, with a rate of 6 breaths/minute or less?
- Is the patient's breathing noisy or laboured (Chaplik and Neafsey 1998)?
- Is the patient's skin cyanosed, does it have a bluish tinge?
- Can high-flow oxygen be started?
- If the patient's breathing is noisy or laboured, have all the interventions on the airway already described been performed as they should be?

Circulation

- When you attempt to palpate a carotid pulse for 10 seconds, can you detect one?
- If there is a pulse, is it notably faster or slower than it was previously?
- If you do not know this, is the patient extremely tachycardic, with a pulse rate of 140 beats/minute (bpm)or more, or profoundly bradycardic, with a pulse rate of ≤40 bpm? Is the pulse rate irregular?
- Is the patient's blood pressure much lower than it was previously (DH 2000)?
- If you are unable to measure a blood pressure, does the patient have signs indicative of hypotension, such as thirst, or dizziness when he or she suddenly stands up (postural hypotension), or a very pale skin and cold fingers and toes, which may indicate poor peripheral circulation?
- When you squeeze the patient's finger for 5 seconds and then release, does it take more than 2 seconds for the skin to go pink, which may indicate a prolonged capillary refill time (Lima and Bakker 2005)?
- Does the skin look dry and wrinkly?
- Has the patient passed no urine for several hours, or has the amount of urine passed been much less than you would expect? Does it average out as less than 30 ml/hour?
- If the patient is pulseless, basic and advanced life support should be initiated as discussed in Chapter 10. If a pulse is present, but the rate is notably slower or faster than you would expect, can you attach the patient to a cardiac monitor or record a 12-lead ECG in order to get more information about the heart?
- If the patient has a low blood pressure or any of the signs that may indicate this, have you laid the patient as flat as he or she can tolerate?

Disability

This can be measured in a number of ways:

- You can record an AVPU score. Is the patient **a**lert, or does he respond to the sound of your **v**oice, or does he respond to **p**ainful stimuli such as squeezing his ear lobe, or is he **u**nresponsive?

- A similar method is the ACDU score. Is the person **a**lert, **c**onfused, **d**rowsy or **u**nresponsive?

Both of these methods have been shown to be reliable ways of measuring deterioration (McNarry and Goldhill 2004).

- If you are recording the patient's score on the Glasgow Coma Scale (GCS) has the total score dropped to ≤8 or by 2 or more points since you last checked it (see www.trauma.org/scores/gcs.html)?

Exposure

- When you expose the patient in such a way as to give you a good view of the torso while maintaining the patient's dignity as far as possible, are there obvious signs of traumatic injury?
- Has the patient got a widespread rash, is there excessive bleeding or is the abdomen tender when you palpate it?
- Has the patient got evidence of burns or been incontinent of faeces or urine, or does the skin feel excessively hot or cold to your touch?

CALLING FOR HELP

When all of these questions related to the ABCDE approach have been answered and all appropriate interventions attempted, make sure that you have called for the appropriate help at the appropriate time. Depending on the patient's situation this might be the cardiac arrest (crash) team, the medical emergency (MET) team, the outreach team or a senior health professional colleague. In the community setting you would need to dial 999 to summon an ambulance. When this assessment of the patient has been made, you may then need to turn your attention to whether the patient's symptoms are a result of myocardial ischaemia or infarction.

THE ECG: WHAT IT IS, WHAT IT DOES

It is useful at this point to consider the role of the ECG in assessing the person with a potential or actual cardiac problem. As part of the circulation assessment described above, it can be useful to attach the patient to a cardiac monitor or to record an ECG, if you have the equipment available. Electrical impulses are generated and conducted throughout the heart, as a result of the chemical ionic changes within cardiac cells. These electrical impulses produce weak electrical currents through the entire body. A graphic record of this can be produced, which is the electrocardiogram, or ECG (Thompson and Webster 2004). An ECG machine contains a galvanometer, effectively a 'moving coil' electric current detector. When a current is passed through a coil in a magnetic field, the coil experiences a movement proportional to the current. If the coil's movement is connected to a coil spring, the amount of deflection of a needle attached to the coil may be proportional to the current passing through the coil. This activity is known as 'meter movement' and is the principle on which early voltmeters and ammeters were based (Nave 2005). In the case of the ECG it allows the changes in electrical potential within the heart to be recorded from the body's surface and for the amplified signal to be recorded on calibrated moving paper or displayed on a screen.

Although electrical impulses are produced throughout the heart, the strongest electrical impulses are produced in specific areas. Generally speaking, conduction begins at the sinoatrial (SA) node, sited near the coronary sinus in the right atrium, and then moves across the atria before being 'picked up' at the atrioventricular (AV) node, sited at the junction of the atria and the ventricles. From there it moves down the bundle of His and into the two bundle branches, right and left, which conduct electricity across the right and left ventricles, respectively. The largest electrical activity occurs in the left ventricle, as the left bundle branch splits into two fascicles, anterior and posterior, which conduct impulses across the left ventricle. As the left ventricle has the largest muscular mass of the four chambers of the heart, it therefore has the largest amount of electrical impulses moving across it. From this it can be seen that this electrical activity, what is sometimes called the wave of depolarisation, moves from right to left across the heart, from SA node to AV node to left ventricle. Sometimes it is said that the wave of conduction moves from the right shoulder to the left foot or from 11 o'clock to 5 o'clock.

Part of the value of the ECG is that it can show the electrical activity of the heart from a number of different angles. The 12 leads of the standard ECG are, in effect, 12 different electrical views or pictures of the heart, normally taken simultaneously. Imagine it as a football game where a goal can be shown from the standard camera angle, but more information about the build-up play and positioning of the players may come from cameras sited behind the goal. Or at a wedding, the official shot of the wedding party may show the bride's father with his arm wrapped protectively around his wife, but only the unofficial picture taken from the side shows that he is concealing an illicit cigarette in his hand. The 12-lead ECG allows us to see the electrical activity of the heart's version of the movement of the players and the hidden cigarette; we see more because we have more angles from which to view.

A further principle of ECG recording is, as a result of the way that the ECG is configured, if the wave of conduction moves towards a particular lead, the lead will show a complex that is predominantly upwards from the baseline when we view it on paper or screen. This is normally known as a positive deflection, and is what we commonly see if we monitor the heart in lead II. Conversely, if we monitor the heart in a lead from which the wave of depolarisation is moving away, this will show a complex that is downwards from the baseline and is thus called a negative deflection (Thompson and Webster

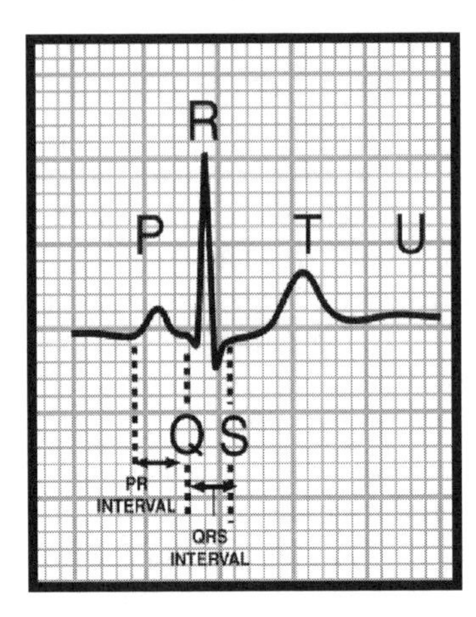

Figure 5.1 A normal ECG complex. (Reproduced by permission of the Resuscitation Council (UK).)

2004). This will normally be seen if we monitor the heart in lead aVR. The other 10 leads will show either a predominantly positive or predominantly negative deflection depending on whether the wave of depolarisation is moving broadly towards them or broadly away from them.

As can be seen in Figure 5.1, the ECG complex can be labelled according to the deflections, which are normally called waves, and the spaces between the start and finish of the various waves, which are normally called intervals. The P wave represents the wave of depolarisation as it is initiated from the SA node. The next wave we see is the Q wave. It is called a Q wave if it is the first deflection after a P wave and if it is negative (downwards). Q waves may be deep, or so shallow as to be no more than a notch, as we see here, or may not be present at all. The first positive (upwards) deflection after a P wave is called an R wave, whether or not it is preceded by a Q wave. Again the size may vary. If the next deflection after an R wave is negative, it is called an S wave. Again these may be large, small or not present. Together these three waves are called the QRS complex and they represent ventricular depolarisation, the wave of conduction as it moves across the ventricles. Remembering what we said earlier about more electrical activity in the larger muscular mass of the left ventricle, the QRS complex normally shows us left ventricular depolarisation; depolarisation is going on simultaneously in the right ventricle, but it is 'drowned out' by the larger electrical depolarisation moving across the left ventricle, so we do not normally see it. As a convention, this part of the ECG tracing is always called the QRS complex, even if one or more of these waves is not be visible. The T wave follows the QRS complex and represents ventricular repolarisation, the time when the ionic activity in the cells of the ventricles is reverting to a state from where it can be ready to depolarise for the next wave of conduction. The U wave is often not seen, but if it is visible it may represent an electrolyte imbalance, such as an unusually low potassium level.

The ECG is recorded by attaching electrodes to the patient that are connected to the ECG machine. In the case of continuous cardiac monitoring, three or five electrodes are usually clipped to adhesive patches, which are then attached to the patient. This form of monitoring is useful for a quick assessment of the patient and for managing cardiac arrhythmias (see Chapter 9). The ECG can also be monitored through defibrillation paddles or adhesive defibrillator pads, although this tends to be done only in emergency situations. If the patient is believed to have ischaemic pain, as well as using one of the monitoring methods described, a 12-lead ECG should be obtained as soon as possible, because the extra 'views' of the heart that it produces are vital in deciding what is happening to the heart and in what particular area.

ASSESSMENT OF MYOCARDIAL ISCHAEMIC PAIN

In addition to the assessment of the patient using the ABCDE approach, one of the critical aspects of assessing the cardiac patient relates to the specific symptom of pain. Accurate assessment of pain allows non-cardiac conditions to be ruled out, and differentiation to be made between stable cardiac conditions and acute coronary syndromes (see Chapters 6 and 7).

The origins of cardiac pain are not fully understood, but there are useful working theories that can help us understand the underlying process and guide the assessment of the patient. There is still some argument as to whether or not the site of ischaemic pain is the coronary arteries themselves, but the generally held view is that the pain comes from the myocardium (Cunningham 2000). A kinin sequence is activated by ischaemia in response to injury to the tissue, whereby bradykinin may activate chemoreceptors in the myocardium. Other mechanisms may be activated by the stretching of the myocardium as a result of ischaemic injury and oedema, causing mechanoreceptors to be activated. Mechanoreceptors may also be activated directly from changes in the coronary arteries (Cunningham 2000). The sensation of pain produced by ischaemia is transferred from the myocardium, via sympathetic fibres that enter the spinal cord at thoracic nerve openings T1–T5, and then transported to the cerebral cortex. The axons from nerves supplying the heart also supply other structures, notably the chest wall, neck, arms, back and jaw. This physiological organisation is important in understanding the phenomenon of *referred ischaemic pain* whereby ischaemic chest pain is accompanied by pain in the arms (normally, but not invariably, the left), neck, back and lower jaw. These areas of the body share the same afferent sympathetic fibres as the myocardium so, when pain impulses from these fibres reach the cerebral cortex, the brain has to 'decide' which area it thinks they are from and send signals to the body accordingly. As the brain 'remembers' pain, if it has felt pain from areas such as the arms, neck, back or jaw in the past, it may signal that pain actually coming from the myocardium is pain from one of these areas (Cunningham 2000).

As myocardial pain is transmitted along the thoracic nerve openings T1–T5 it follows that it will be 'mistaken' for pain only from other areas that share these pathways; ischaemic pain is bounded by these areas because the supplying nerves are seldom above spinal nerve C3 or below spinal nerve T6. Any shared pain pathways running beyond these boundaries will not be perceived as referred ischaemic pain. In practice, this means that referred ischaemic pain is not normally perceived below the umbilical area or above the lower jaw. It should be remembered, of course, that this assumes that we believe that myocardial pain is coming from either the coronary arteries or the myocardium. If this is felt as pain spreading across and around the whole of the chest, this too is a referral from the original site of the pain, although this is regarded as 'classic' myocardial ischaemic pain (MIP) rather than 'referred' pain.

In relation to specific disorders, MIP refers to pain that is caused by ischaemia and accompanies stable angina, acute coronary syndromes and myocardial infarction in its various presentations. This pain is typically described as being present in the chest, being retrosternal (i.e. behind the breast bone) and perhaps radiating to the back, neck, arms and lower jaw. The pain is often described by sufferers using terms such as 'like a tight band round my chest', crushing', 'pressing' or 'heavy', or 'like someone sitting on my chest'. Not infrequently sufferers will describe it as being 'like an elephant sittting on my chest' which, leaving aside how they would know what this felt like, gives a graphic illustration of the idea of an extreme crushing weight. The pain may be associated with feelings of nausea and actual vomiting, particularly if the inferoposterior wall (i.e. the bottom and the back) of the heart is the main site of the ischaemic pain, because the vagal nerve may be involved here and vagal reflexes producing bradycardias and hypotension may manifest themselves as dizziness or fainting. The person with the pain often sweats and the skin is pale and feels clammy to the touch.

Importantly, the pain is usually continuous, and changing the position or taking in a deep breath does not usually alter the character and severity of the pain. It may come on either suddenly or gradually, and it may be associated with anger, stress or exercise, but it may also have come on at rest and can wake the person from sleep. Sometimes, when describing the pain, people will make a circular motion of their hand across the front of the chest or move a hand back and forth across the chest, indicating how widespread the pain is. Sometimes a patient will clench a fist and press it towards the breastbone. This is called Levine's sign and can be regarded as a useful marker for ischaemic pain, along with other signs such as a flat hand placed on the chest, indicating the heaviness of the sensation, and both hands placed on the chest with the fingers pointing at each other and then pulled apart distally. One study has suggested that these are accurate predictors of whether chest pain is ischaemic in origin (Edmondstone 1995). Confusingly, the pain is sometimes called 'indigestion like'. The ischaemic pain of a heart attack is often described as being the worst pain that the patient has ever experienced, although mothers will sometimes say that the pain of childbirth is more acute. Importantly, however, other subgroups, including people with diabetes and elderly people, may have much less severe pain presentations.

It can be useful to consider ischaemic pain negatively, i.e. to think about ways in which the pain does not usually manifest itself. It is rare for ischaemic pain to be described as 'sharp' or 'stabbing'. A rider needs to be added here that sometimes people will use 'stabbing' to mean 'extremely severe' rather than 'knife like'. This is an area where more than most it is vital to be clear what our patients are telling us. If a patient points directly at an area of pain in the chest with one finger, this is unlikely to be MIP. This becomes less likely still if, on further questioning, the patient describes the area of the pain as being smaller than the area covered by the end of a finger (Cunningham 2000). If the pain changes in intensity when the person alters position, or breathes deeply in or out, then it is unlikely to be ischaemic pain.

ECG EVIDENCE OF MYOCARDIAL INFARCTION

The ECG may be helpful in deciding if the pain is the result of myocardial ischaemia. Sometimes it may accurately predict a myocardial ischaemic event. The diagnostic triad of the World Health Organization (WHO) for a myocardial infarction (MI) is typical MIP, ST elevation of 2 mm or more in two limb consecutive limb leads or three consecutive pre-cordial leads, and biochemical markers such as a positive troponin blood test. The WHO considerered that any two of these three tests is enough for a positive diagnosis of an MI (WHO Expert Committee 1959). More recently, guidelines have been published that put more emphasis on symptoms and ECG criteria in an attempt to allow diagnosis to be made as soon as possible, so that effective management can begin immediately. Although biochemical markers such as creatine kinase (CK) or troponin should be used formally to diagnose an MI, they may well take too long to allow urgent treatment (Hahn and Chandler 2006).

Guidelines from the European Society of Cardiology and the American College of Cardiology recommend that a diagnosis can be made if MIP is present and accompanied by ST elevation in two or more contiguous leads (i.e. leads that are next to each other in the way that they view the heart, such as II and aVF or V3 and V4) of at least 2 mm in V2 and V3 and 1 mm in all other leads, assuming that these are all new changes (Alpert et al. 2000). More recent guidelines have recommended that the measurement should be 1 mm of ST elevation in two or more contiguous leads, although Antman et al. (2004) recognise that this would reduce the specificity of the ECG as a diagnostic tool in certain situations. This ambiguity apart, what we are looking for is ST elevation in at least two leads looking at the same area of myocardium, measured from the J point, the part of the ECG complex where the QRS complex meets the ST segment (Wagner 2001) (Figure 5.2).

The first QRS complex in Figure 5.2 shows the ST segment to be isoelectric, i.e. on the same level as the baseline between the P wave and the QRS and after the T wave. The second complex shows ST elevation, where the QRS complex seems to merge into the T wave, without returning to the baseline first. The ST segment represents the period of time during which the ventricles are depolarised, i.e. when the electrical changes have spent themselves across the ventricles. As there is usually no electrical activity during this period of time, the ST segment is commonly isoelectric (Wagner 2001).

The ECG in Figure 5.3 shows clear ST elevation of several millimetres in leads V2–V5 and leads I and aVL. Given that this patient also had MIP, the diagnosis of an MI was easily made. Leads V1 and V2 also show unusually

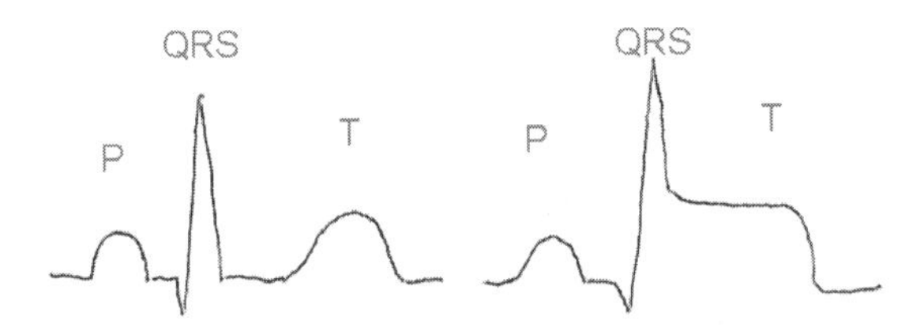

Figure 5.2 ST elevation.

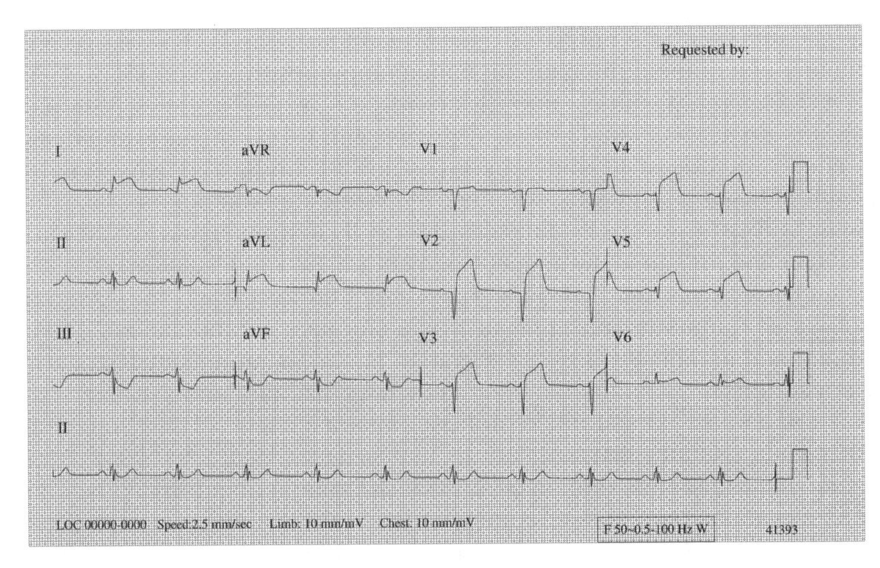

Figure 5.3 ECG evidence of myocardial infarction.

deep Q waves, an indicator that some permanent damage has been done to the heart. ST elevation will eventually resolve, but will often leave Q waves, which may be permanent. The V leads 'look' at the front of the heart, so this can be called an 'anterior' MI. The changes described in leads I and aVL indicate that the lateral aspect of the heart is also involved. Leads I and aVL show a similar region of the heart to V5 and V6, but higher up; thus they are sometimes called the 'high lateral' leads, and an ECG that shows ST elevation in V5 and V6 as well as I and aVL can be said to be showing an 'anterolateral' infarction. Had these changes been in leads II, III or aVF, leads that look at the underside of the heart, this would have been an 'inferior' MI.

Interestingly, this ECG does show changes in the inferior leads, where the ST segment seems to be depressed rather than elevated. ST depression in the absence of ST elevation is often a sign of reversible ischaemia (Smith and Kampine 1990) and may be present in chronic stable angina. In such circumstances, when the pain resolves, the ECG changes will do likewise. In this example, the inferior changes may be an example of so-called 'reciprocal' changes; this means that in effect the ST depression in these leads is a mirror image of the ST elevation in the anterior leads (Parale et al. 2004). The other principal site of infarction is the posterior wall of the heart. Given that there are no leads that 'look' directly at the back of the heart, we must infer what area is involved examining the leads that 'look' at the front of the heart: V1 and V2. Instead of there being ST elevation and Q waves, as we would see in an anterior MI, a posterior MI may show ST depression and an unusually prominent R wave in these leads (Bareiss et al. 1989).

REASONS TO BE CAREFUL

Part of the difficulty in assessing whether the person in front of you is undergoing an ischaemic event comes from the fact that there are a number of other conditions that can mimic MIP to a greater or lesser extent. Some of this is a result of poor history taking on the part of the initial assessor. Over the years, I have at times been bemused by people referred to coronary care units with a provisional diagnosis of 'chest pain – ?MI' who then turn out to be having pain as diversely spread as groin pain (correctly diagnosed as an inguinal hernia) and headache (which, unsurprisingly, proved to be a migraine). Once the reported symptom of 'sudden onset of central chest pain' turned out to have been caused when the patient had been hit by a train; on another occasion this phrase was used to describe the pain of a man who had been working under his car when it fell off the jack!

Nevertheless, sometimes errors are made because this is a difficult area. One of the ways in which we can minimise errors is to use the ECG as effectively as possible. It has been shown that so-called 'atypical' presentations of chest pain are as likely to have typical ischaemic ECG changes as people with nic pain and that around 1 person in 11 experiencing an acute coronary may have no chest pain at all (Brieger et al. 2004).

ie ECG is unhelpful, we ensure that we can assess the pain as effectively as possible. Generally, it is useful to assume initially that chest pain may be ischaemic in origin and then try to eliminate this as a diagnosis, because an MI will generally be more problematic and more in need of early management than other possible causative factors. Ischaemia is frequently dismissed as indigestion by both clinicians and patients although up to 40% of these people may be having an MI (Simpson et al. 1984). A patient may not wonder why indigestion seems much worse than normal and is not relieved by the usual antacid, but you should. In general, the maxim 'when a young man complains of his heart, look to his stomach, when an old man complains of his stomach, look to his heart', although unscientific, may be very useful (Simpson et al. 1984).

Musculoskeletal pains can frequently mimic ischaemia, even including radiation from the chest to arms (Frobert et al. 1999). In general, if the pain is significantly worse on movement, it is unlikely to be ischaemic in origin. Pulmonary causes of chest pain may mimic ischaemia and are most probably the result of bacterial chest infections; as such they are generally less problematic. A very small percentage may be extremely dangerous conditions such as pulmonary embolism (PE) or acute aortic aneurysm dissection (Kohn et al. 2005). PE should be suspected if the person has recently had lack of mobility, whether as a result of illness or injury or social factors such as long journeys. The ECG may be helpful in diagnosing PE, with sinus tachycardia being a fairly common sign along with inverted T waves in the chest leads (Ferrari et al. 1997), but the so-called classic sign of a deep S wave in lead I and a Q wave and inverted T wave in lead III (S1 Q3 T3) is just as likely to be seen in people without a PE and have led some to conclude that the ECG is fairly unhelpful in diagnosing PE (Rodger et al. 2000). The pain of aortic dissection is often described by people experiencing it as 'tearing' and diagnosis may be more easily made if a difference in blood pressure can be discerned between the right and left arm, although this finding may well be prevalent in someone without aortic dissection (Singer and Hollander 1996). Generally speaking, if the pain seems to be worse when the patient breathes in deeply, it is likely that the cause is in the lung rather than the heart.

Pericarditis may be mistaken for ischaemic pain, whether it is of acute viral or bacterial onset or secondary to cardiac surgery or a heart attack. The ECG in pericarditis may show widespread ST elevation that is 'saddle shaped', i.e. concave, rather than convex, as is normally the case in an MI. In addition a pericardial rub, a dry scratchy heart sound, can sometimes be heard (Ross and Grauer 2004, Carter and Brooks 2005). Again, this pain may change on movement; it can be useful to lay the patient flat and then sit him or her up. The pain is likely to be relieved as the patient sits up. Pericarditis is discussed in greater detail in Chapter 12.

CONCLUSION

Assessment of the cardiac patient is best achieved by a systematic approach. First assess the patient using the ABCDE method, and then assess the character of the pain that the patient is experiencing. A good knowledge of the ECG will help enormously in deciding if the patient's pain is ischaemic in origin. If the symptoms and the ECG suggest an MI, it is essential that appropriate help be summoned to allow for rapid assessment and treatment by a clinician able to manage this condition.

REFERENCES

Alpert JS, Thygesen K Antman E et al. (2000) Myocardial infarction redefined – a consensus document of the Joint European Society of Cardiology/American College of Cardiology Committee for the redefinition of myocardial infarction. *Journal of the American College of Cardiology* **36**: 959–69.

Antman EM, Anbe DT, Armstron PW et al. (2004) ACC/AHA guidelines for the management of patients with ST elevation myocardial infarction: part of the American College of Cardiology/American Heart Association Task force on Practice Guidelines (Committee to revise the 1999 guidelines for the management of patients with acute myocardial infarction). *Circulation* **110**: 82–292.

Bareiss P, Rochoux G, Roul G et al. (1989) Isolated ST-segment depression in precordial leads V2 to V4. An early electrocardiographic sign of posterolateral myocardial infarction *Annales de Cardiologie et d'Angéiologie* **38**: 265–8.

Bein B, Scholz J (2005) Supraglottic airway devices. *Best Practice and Research. Clinical Anaesthesiology* **19**: 581–93.

Brieger D, Eagle KA, Goodman SG et al. (2004) Acute coronary syndromes without chest pain, an underdiagnosed and undertreated high risk group, insights from the Global Registry of Acute Coronary Events. *Chest* **126**: 461–9.

Carter T, Brooks CA (2005) Pericarditis: inflammation or infarction? *Journal of Cardiovascular Nursing* **20**: 239–44.

Chaplik S, Neafsey P (1998) Pre-existing variables and outcome of cardiac arrest resuscitation in hospitalized patients. *Dimensions of Critical Care Nursing* **17**: 200–7.

Cunningham S (2000) Pathophysiology of myocardial ischemia and infarction. In: Woods S, Froelicher E, Motzer S (eds), *Cardiac Nursing*, 4th edn. Philadelphia: Lippincott.

Department of Health (2000) *Comprehensive Critical Care: A review of adult critical care services*. London: Department of Health.

Edmondstone W (1995) Cardiac chest pain: does body language help the diagnosis? *British Medical Journal* **311**: 1660–1.

Ferrari E, Imbert A, Chevalier T et al. (1997) The electrocardiogram in pulmonary embolism: predictive value of negative T waves in precordial leads – 80 case reports. *Chest* **11**: 537–43.

Frobert O, Fossgreen J, Sondergaard-Petersen J et al. (1999) Musculo-skeletal pathology in patients with angina pectoris and normal coronary angiograms. *Journal of Internal Medicine* **245**: 237–46.

Hahn S, Chandler C (2006) Diagnosis and management of ST elevation myocardial infarction: A review of the recent literature and practice guidelines. *Mount Sinai Journal of Medicine* **73**: 1469–81.

Harrison GA, Jaques TC, Kilborn G et al. (2005) The prevalence of recordings of signs of critical conditions and emergency responses in hospital wards – the SOCCER study. *Resuscitation* **65**: 147–57.

Jaworski CA (2002) Advances in emergent airway management. *Current Sports Medicine Reports* **1**(3): 133–40.

Kohn M, Kwan E, Gupta M, Tabas J (2005) Prevalence of acute myocardial infarction and other serious diagnoses in patients presenting to an urban emergency department with chest pain. *Journal of Emergency Medicine* **29**: 383–90.

Lima A, Bakker J (2005) Noninvasive monitoring of peripheral perfusion. *Intensive Care Medicine* **31**: 1316–26.

McArthur-Rouse F (2001) Critical care outreach services and early warning scoring systems: a review of the literature. *Journal of Advanced Nursing* **36**: 696–704.

McNarry A, Goldhill D (2004). Simple bedside assessment of level of consciousness: comparison of two simple assessment scales with the Glasgow Coma scale. *Anaesthesia* **59**(1): 34–7.

McQuillan P, Pilkington S, Allan A et al. (1998) Confidential inquiry into quality of care before admission to intensive care. *British Medical Journal* **316**: 1853–8.

Nave R (2005) *Hyperphysics*. Department of Physics and Astronomy, Georgia State University. Available from hyperphysics.phy-astr.gsu.edu/hbase/hph.html.

Parale GP, Kulkarni PM, Khade SK (2004) Importance of reciprocal leads in acute myocardial infarction. *Journal of Association of Physicians in India* **52**: 376–9.

Resuscitation Council (UK) (2006) *Advanced Life Support*, 5th edn. London: Resuscitation Council (UK).

Rodger M, Makropoulos D, Turek M et al. (2000) Diagnostic value of the electrocardiogram in suspected pulmonary embolism. *American Journal of Cardiology* **86**: 807–9.

Ross AM, Grauer SE (2004) Acute pericarditis. Evaluation and treatment of infectious and other causes. *Postgraduate Medicine* **115**(3): 67–75.

Simpson FG, Kay J, Aber CP (1984) Chest pain – indigestion or impending heart attack? *Postgraduate Medical Journal* **60**: 338–40.

Singer AJ, Hollander JE (1996) Blood pressure. Assessment of interarm differences. *Archives of Internal Medicine* **156**: 2005–8.

Smith JJ, Kampine JP (1990) *Circulatory Physiology – the essentials*, 3rd edn. Baltimore, MD: Williams & Wilkins.

Smith A, Wood J (1998) Can some in-hospital cardio-respiratory arrests be prevented? A prospective survey. *Resuscitation* **37**: 133–7.

Thompson D, Webster R (2004) *Caring for the Cardiac Patient.* Oxford: Butterworth-Heinemann.

Wagner G (2001) *Marriott's Practical Electrocardiography*, 10th edn. Philadelphia: Lippincott, Williams & Wilkins.

World Health Organization Expert Committee (1959) *Hypertension and Coronary Heart Disease: Classification and criteria for epidemiological studies*. Geneva: WHO.

6 Coronary heart disease: stable angina

TOM QUINN

Angina was first described by Heberden (1772) over three centuries ago:

> They who are afflicted with it, are seized while they are walking (more especially if it be uphill and soon after eating) with a painful and most disagreeable sensation in the breast, which seems as if it would extinguish life, if it were to increase or to continue; but the moment they stand still, all this uneasiness vanishes.

Heberden's definition is still in widespread use (Abrams 2005, Abrams and Thadani 2005, Thompson and Webster 2005). The predictable and reproducible symptoms described above result from inadequate coronary perfusion in response to increases in myocardial oxygen requirements. One or more major coronary arteries in the patient with angina are usually obstructed (stenosed) by at least 70%.

When symptoms are wholly and predictably related to exertion and completely reversible with cessation of physical activity or simple treatment with sublingual nitrate, angina is said to be 'stable'. Recent-onset, prolonged or frequent symptoms, and those occurring at rest, are termed 'unstable angina' and are discussed in Chapter 7. Angina symptoms can be accentuated by conditions such as hypertension, anaemia and thyrotoxicosis.

The condition is not benign, particularly in the weeks following onset of initial symptoms where there is high risk of progression to acute coronary syndrome with 10% of patients with new-onset angina dying or having a myocardial infarction (MI), and a further 20% undergoing a revascularisation procedure within the first year of presentation (Gandhi et al. 1995) However, most patients with chronic stable angina have a favourable long-term prognosis in the absence of high-risk characteristics such as previous MI, diabetes, advanced age or hypertension (Hjemdahl et al. 2005).

Cardiac Care: An Introduction for Healthcare Professionals. Edited by David Barrett, Mark Gretton and Tom Quinn
© 2006 John Wiley & Sons Ltd

PATHOPHYSIOLOGY AND BURDEN OF DISEASE

Angina is a common condition in the UK, with the British Heart Foundation (BHF 2005) estimating 181 000 new cases of angina in British men and 160 000 in British women – a total of 341 000 people presenting each year. Incidence rises with age and is higher in men than in women. In the UK just under two million people are estimated to be living with, or to have had a diagnosis of, angina (BHF 2005). The published data are for people under the age of 75 years and are therefore likely to underestimate the burden of this condition significantly in an ageing population. Based on data from community registers, exertional angina is considered to be the most common first presentation of coronary heart disease (CHD): less than 14% of CHD patients present first with sudden death, and over half of men and two-thirds of women have preserved myocardium (i.e. have not sustained an MI) on first presentation (Sutcliffe et al. 2003).

Certain groups within society appear to be at higher risk of developing CHD and therefore angina. These issues have been discussed further in Chapter 1.

The burden of angina is also reflected in increased use of medicines and procedures (diagnostic coronary angiography, percutaneous intervention and coronary bypass grafting) across the UK. The use of evidence-based treatments has increased since the publication of the National Service Framework (NSF) for CHD in England (Department of Health or DH 2000) and similar policies in Wales (National Assembly for Wales 2001) and Scotland (Scottish Executive Health Department 2002). The widespread introduction of rapid access chest pain clinics (RACPCs), discussed below, has facilitated prompt referral and specialist assessment of large numbers of patients with new-onset chest pain.

Stewart et al. (2003) have estimated that there are 634 000 primary care consultations for angina each year, with the overall cost of caring for angina patients consuming around 1% of the total NHS budget.

PATHOPHYSIOLOGY

The usual cause of anginal symptoms resulting from myocardial ischaemia is an imbalance between myocardial oxygen supply and demand. In most patients with stable angina, the underlying cause is severe narrowing (70% or more) of one or more coronary arteries as a result of atherosclerotic changes within the vessel.

Atherosclerosis is a complex progressive condition associated with dynamic interactions of blood elements, alterations in blood flow and vessel wall abnormalities (Quinn et al. 2002). Atherosclerosis begins in childhood and progresses through young adulthood to form the lesions that cause CHD. These preclinical lesions are associated with CHD risk factors in young people (McMahan et al. 2005). The atherosclerotic process is characterised by the proliferation of smooth muscle cells and accumulation of elevated white lesions ('plaque') in the vessel intima. Plaques comprise a lipid core and fibrous outer layer. Plaques with high lipid content are more vulnerable to rupture.

Emerging evidence strongly suggests that CHD is a manifestation of a chronic inflammatory response to injury or infection, and not solely the result of lipid deposition (Chilton 2004). Injury or infection can disrupt normal endothelial function and initiate formation of atherosclerotic lesions ('fatty streaks'), consisting of macrophages and T cells embedded in thin layers of lipids in the arterial wall (Ross 1999). As atherosclerosis progresses, plaque is deposited external to the lumen, allowing the diameter to be maintained – a phenomenon demonstrated by intravascular ultrasound studies of the coronary arteries and known as the Glagov effect or 'positive remodelling' (Schoenhagen et al. 2000, Abrams 2005).

As atherosclerosis worsens over time, however, the plaque may encroach into the vessel lumen, resulting in obstruction of blood flow and giving rise to exertional angina symptoms. In addition, disorders of the endothelial vasodilator function within the coronary artery or arteries result in reduced ability to vasodilate (which would increase intracoronary blood flow) and instead tending towards vasoconstriction, further reducing flow during exercise and other stimuli (Halcox et al. 2002). In acute coronary syndromes, the degree of obstruction is less important than the so-called 'vulnerability' of the plaque: erosion or ulceration of a fibrous cap (which may not have been obstructive and was therefore clinically silent before the event) results in intraluminal thrombus, leading to sudden death or infarction.

Myocardial ischaemia results from coronary blood flow that is inadequate to meet myocardial oxygen demand. As myocardial oxygen supply is generally determined by coronary blood flow, reduced flow resulting from an obstructed vessel causes symptoms once demand increases. Myocardial oxygen demand depends primarily on heart rate, the force of myocardial contraction and left ventricular wall tension. Most coronary blood flow occurs during diastole.

SYMPTOMS AND PRESENTATION

Descriptive information from the patient with chest pain is crucial to the clinician, whether nurse, doctor or ambulance paramedic, undertaking the initial assessment. The quality, location, duration and presence of any triggers, or aggravating (or indeed relieving) factors, should all be elucidated. This initial information can support the clinician in classifying chest pain as typical or atypical angina, or non-cardiac chest pain, and in distinguishing between suspected stable angina and an acute coronary syndrome. The initial assessment should also include assessment of risk factors for cardiovascular disease such as smoking, hyperlipidaemia, diabetes mellitus, hypertension and family history of premature CHD (Snow et al. 2004). The presence of any other conditions (e.g. anaemia, thyroid dysfunction, valvular disorders) that might precipitate anginal symptoms should be excluded. Non-cardiac causes of chest pain (e.g. aortic dissection, pulmonary embolism, chest infection, local trauma) should also be considered.

Descriptions of anginal symptoms have been reported by Philpott et al. (2001) to differ between men and women, with women describing more throat, neck or jaw pain than men. Women also gave more accounts than men of breathlessness and other symptoms. The prognostic significance of dyspnoea in patients referred for cardiac stress testing has recently been highlighted by Abidov et al. (2005). Self-reported dyspnoea identified a subgroup of otherwise asymptomatic patients at increased risk of death from cardiac and other causes. Key features of chest pain caused by CHD are (Fox 2005):

- Family history of CHD (male first-degree relative <55 years of age; female <60 years)
- Hyperlipidaemia
- Hypertension
- Diabetes mellitus
- Typical pain location (central) and radiation (to left arm and throat/jaw)
- Tight, constricting in character
- Duration >5 minutes
- Aggravated by exertion
- Relieved by rest (or nitrates).

The Canadian Cardiovascular Society have published a widely used classification tool for assessing the functional status angina of patients (Sangareddi et al. 2004) as shown in Table 6.1.

Table 6.1 Canadian Cardiovascular Society functional classification tool

Class	Definition
I	No angina with ordinary physical activity (e.g. walking, climbing stairs). Angina occurs with strenuous or prolonged exertion
II	Early onset limitation of ordinary activity (e.g. walking rapidly or walking more than two blocks; climbing stairs rapidly or more than one flight); angina may be worse after meals, in cold temperatures or with emotional stress
III	Marked limitation of ordinary activity
IV	Inability to carry out any physical activity without chest discomfort. Angina occurs during rest

From Sangareddi et al. (2004).

INVESTIGATION AND MANAGEMENT

Initial investigations include vital signs and a detailed physical examination, together with a resting 12-lead electrocardiogram (ECG), often found to be normal in the absence of symptoms. Venous blood should be taken for full blood count (FBC) to exclude anaemia, thyroid function and urea and electrolytes (U&Es). The clinical utility of cardiac biomarkers remains uncertain in the non-acute setting (Abrams 2005). Patients presenting in primary care settings (e.g. general practice or 'walk-in' centre) who have symptoms suggesting an acute coronary syndrome (rest pain, associated dyspnoea, vomiting, pallor, etc.) should be referred immediately to the emergency ambulance service by a 999 call (see Chapter 7). This chapter focuses on patients thought to have stable angina.

Adults with typical or atypical chest pain – especially in the presence of risk factors for cardiovascular disease – should undergo exercise tolerance testing. In England, the NSF has ensured the availability of an RACPC in most, if not all, general hospitals so that patients who are thought by the GP or emergency department to have new-onset stable angina, can undergo specialist assessment, including an exercise tolerance test, within 2 weeks of referral. Secondary prevention with aspirin to reduce the risk of adverse events such as an acute MI should begin immediately without waiting for the RACPC appointment. The concept and functions of an RACPC are discussed in more detail below.

RISK STRATIFICATION

Risk stratification is used widely in primary prevention of cardiovascular diseases as discussed in Chapter 3. A score for identifying stable angina patients who may be at increased risk of serious adverse events, including MI, stroke or all-cause mortality, has been proposed by Clayton et al. (2005). The score is based on 16 routinely available variables including age, smoking, diabetes and left ventricular function; patients in the highest tenth of scores had ten times the risk of serious adverse events of patients in the lowest tenth (Clayton et al. 2005). Whether this proposed risk score will be helpful, in clinical practice, in identifying patients for revascularisation, remains subject to further research (Terkelsen and Vach 2005). In one randomised controlled trial comparing nicorandil with placebo in over 5000 patients with stable angina, the Canadian Cardiovascular Society score and a history of previous MI were the strongest risk factors for adverse events (IONA Study Group 2005). High resting heart rate has recently been described as a predictor for total and cardiovascular mortality, independent of other risk factors in patients with coronary disease (Diaz et al. 2005).

KEY GOALS IN STABLE ANGINA: SYMPTOM CONTROL AND RISK REDUCTION

Key goals in treating the patient with stable angina include symptom control and risk reduction. Lifestyle advice, particularly on smoking cessation and exercise, together with lipid lowering and other medication, plays a major role; there is considerable evidence that this dual approach may reduce progression of atherosclerosis and stabilise plaque in patients with chronic stable angina (Gibbons et al. 2003, Nissen et al. 2004). Regular exercise can reduce the frequency of anginal symptoms and improve endothelial function (Gielen et al. 2001, Gibbons et al. 2003). The use of aspirin reduces cardiovascular morbidity and mortality in patients with stable angina (Juul-Moller et al. 1992). Statins are also known to reduce coronary event rates and are recommended for use in patients with established CHD or in those at risk (DH 2000).

Drugs used to treat patients with angina are collectively termed 'anti-anginals' and consist primarily of three groups – nitrates, β blockers and calcium channel blockers. Although none of these drugs has been proved to prolong life or to prevent MI, they do improve functional performance, increasing exercise capacity without symptoms. No single class of drugs has been shown to be superior in terms of anti-anginal effect than the others. It is therefore considered acceptable to start patients on any of the three groups as initial therapy (Abrams 2005). Cardiac medications are discussed in more detail in Chapter 13.

RAPID ACCESS CHEST PAIN CLINICS

The NSF sets out plans to establish RACPCs in hospitals across England to facilitate rapid specialist assessment of patients with new-onset chest pain thought by the referring GP to be stable angina (DH 2000). This model of care has been successful in improving access for this group of patients, enabling high-risk patients to be identified and managed, and those without significant CHD to be reassured and discharged back to the care of their GP. The concept of rapid access for chest pain patients is not new: several observational studies were published before the NSF and helped to shape the policy (Norell et al. 1992, Jain et al. 1997, Newby et al. 1998).

Typically, patients are referred to an RACPC using protocols agreed between primary and secondary care under the aegis of the local CHD implementation group or cardiac network. Most areas have developed and agreed standardised proforma to facilitate referral and reduce delay. The key information required from a referring GP might include (alongside basic demographic information such as name, age, date of birth) symptom characteristics and duration, any risk factors for CHD and exclusion of contraindications to exercise testing (e.g. impaired mobility, aortic stenosis). A resting 12-lead ECG commonly forms part of the referral process, not to exclude CHD – a normal ECG does not rule out important coronary disease (Norell et al. 1992) – but to provide a baseline and to exclude bundle-branch block (BBB), left ventricular hypertrophy or pacemaker activity, which would preclude analysis of an exercise tolerance test. In many cases the GP is also asked to send venous blood for analysis of a patient's lipid profile, FBC, etc. Local protocols should emphasise that the RACPC is not the appropriate route for referral of patients with suspected acute coronary syndromes (for whom a 999 ambulance is required) or those with known CHD already under the care of the cardiology department.

Tertiary cardiac centres running an RACPC service may, however, provide 'slots' within the RACPC for assessment of patients with recurrent symptoms, including those who have undergone interventional procedures, although the latter should arguably be seen as emergency cases. Referrals are commonly 'screened' by a specialist cardiac nurse or middle-grade doctor to ensure that RACPC attendance is appropriate; patients are then contacted by telephone or in writing to offer an appointment. Increasingly, such appointments may be made electronically from the GP surgery. Patients are provided with information about what to expect during the RACPC visit and what to wear to facilitate exercise testing, and advised about medication (e.g. whether or not to continue taking β blockers).

On arrival at the RACPC patients undergo initial assessment of vital signs and a resting 12-lead ECG; urinalysis and weight may be included. A baseline clinical assessment – history and clinical examination – is undertaken by the specialist nurse or doctor, depending on local arrangements. Bloods may be sent for FBC, U&Es, glucose and lipids, if this has not already done by the referring GP. If the history is suggestive of angina, and the patient is stable and able to exercise, then an exercise tolerance test is performed. The exercise tolerance test is the most widely used non-invasive test in the early assessment of the patient with suspected stable angina and is extremely safe, with a mortality of 1 in 10 000 tests. Competencies for the safe supervision of patients undergoing an exercise tolerance test have been published (Rodgers et al. 2000). The interpretation of an exercise test should be undertaken by a suitably competent and experienced practitioner – the detailed conduct of an exercise test and the application of Bayes' theorem (the post-test likelihood of CHD depends on the result of the test together with the pre-test likelihood of CHD) are outside the scope of this chapter.

A negative exercise test in a patient with a low–moderate probability of CHD effectively eliminates the likelihood of significant coronary disease and patients can usually be reassured and the search for other causes of their symptoms can start (Fox 2005). The key, as previously stated, is evaluation of the test results in combination with the whole clinical picture by a suitably competent professional.

For those patients in whom the exercise test result is equivocal or where the patient has been unable to perform the physical exertion required (because of pre-existing illness such as asthma or disability such as arthritis, etc.) additional 'functional tests' such as stress echocardiography, myocardial perfusion imaging or magnetic resonance imaging (MRI) may be required. In cases where these tests are negative the risk of a major cardiac event in ensuing years is below 1% (Fox 2005).

A small minority of patients attending an RACPC will have an acute coronary syndrome and will require immediate admission to A&E or a cardiac care unit (CCU). If thrombolytic treatment is indicated for an ST elevation MI (STEMI) in a patient attending an RACPC, this should be administered before transfer if possible; where facilities exist for immediate percutaneous coronary intervention (PCI) this is the preferred strategy.

The needs and experiences of patients attending an RACPC have been studied by Price et al. (2005), who reported that patients want to be reassured, know and understand what is causing their symptoms, and feel able to help themselves. Additional oral and written information and advice can be effective in informing patients about their condition, raising awareness of risk factors for CHD and promoting lifestyle changes (Price et al. 2005). Patients who have a cardiac cause for their pain excluded continue to report symptoms, uncertainty and disability (Mayou et al. 1994, Goodacre et al. 2001).

ANGIOGRAPHY

Coronary angiography remains the diagnostic gold standard for CHD patients and is indicated in patients with poorly controlled symptoms, abnormal stress test results (especially where there is significant ST segment shift on the ECG), significant left ventricular wall-motion abnormalities on echocardiography or substantial defects on myocardial perfusion imaging. Occasionally, angiography may be required for patients who have atypical chest pain or inconclusive exercise tolerance tests. This procedure is explored in Chapter 14.

REVASCULARISATION

Revascularisation with PCI or coronary artery bypass (CAB) grafting should be considered in patients who do not respond adequately to anti-anginal medical therapy, those who lead an active lifestyle, patients with a large ischaemic burden and those with severe disease, especially if there is left ventricular dysfunction (Abrams and Thadani 2005). Symptoms are relieved in 80–90% of patients undergoing revascularisation but, compared with medical treatment alone, revascularisation does not appear to prolong life or reduce the risk of an acute MI (Abrams 2005). Long-term comparisons of outcome in patients having either PCI or CAB, particularly in the era of drug-eluting stents, are unclear (Babapulle et al. 2004, Hill et al. 2004). Chapters 14 and 15 provide more information about PCI and CAB.

SELF-MANAGEMENT – THE ANGINA PLAN

Many patients with stable angina report a poor quality of life, with raised levels of anxiety and depression (Lewin 1999). A randomised trial of the 'angina plan' concluded that psychological, symptomatic and functional status were improved by a cognitive–behavioural disease management programme in patients with newly diagnosed angina (Lewin et al. 2002).

CONCLUSION

Angina pectoris affects an estimated 2 million people in the UK and results in impaired quality of life, consumes high levels of health service resources and, although the long-term outlook appears favourable in 'low-risk' patients, carries a high early mortality. Services for this group of patients have improved since publication of the NSF (DH 2000), with better access to specialised assessment and revascularisation where required. More research is needed to determine the optimal management strategy for angina patients, including not only medical treatments but also improvement in quality of life through appropriate use of 'self-help' programmes.

REFERENCES

Abidov A, Rosanski A, Hachamovitch R et al. (2005) Prognostic significance of dyspnea in patients referred for cardiac stress testing. *New England Journal of Medicine* **353**: 1889–98.

Abrams J (2005) Chronic stable angina. *New England Journal of Medicine* 352: 2524–2533.

Abrams J, Thadani U (2005) Therapy of stable angina pectoris. The uncomplicated patient. *Circulation* **112**: e255–9.

Babapulle M, Joseph L, Belisle P et al. (2004) A hierarchical Bayesian meta-analysis of randomised clinical trials of drug eluting stents. *Lancet* **364**: 583–91.

British Heart Foundation (2005) *Coronary Heart Disease Statistics*. Available from www.heartstats.org.

Chilton R (2004) Pathophysiology of coronary heart disease: a brief review. *Journal of the American Osteopathic Association* **104**: S5–8.

Clayton T, Lubsen J, Pocock S et al. (2005) Risk score for predicting death, myocardial infarction, and stroke in patients with stable angina, based on a large randomised trial cohort of patients. *British Medical Journal* **331**: 869–72.

Department of Health (2000) *National Service Framework for Coronary Heart Disease.* London: Department of Health.

Diaz A, Bourassa M, Guertin M et al. (2005) Long term prognostic value of resting heart rate in patients with suspected or proven coronary artery disease. *European Heart Journal* **26**: 967–74.

Fox K (2005) Investigation and management of chest pain. *Heart* **91**: 105–10.

Gandhi M, Lampe F, Wood D (1995) Incidence, clinical characteristics and short-term prognosis of angina pectoris. *Heart* **73**: 193–8.

Gibbons RJ, Abrams J, Chatterjee K et al. (2003) ACC/AHA 2002 guideline update for the management of patients with chronic stable angina – summary article: a report of the American College of Cardiology/American Heart Association Task Force on Practice Guidelines (Committee on the Management of Patients With Chronic Stable Angina). *Circulation* **107**: 149–58.

Gielen S, Schuler G, Hambrecht R (2001) Exercise training in coronary artery disease and coronary vasomotion. *Circulation* **103**: E1–6.

Goodacre S, Mason S, Arnold J et al. (2001) Psychologic morbidity and health related quality of life of patients assessed in a chest pain observation unit. *Annals of Emergency Medicine* **38**: 369–76.

Halcox J, Schenke W, Zalos G et al. (2002) Prognostic value of coronary vascular endothelial dysfunction. *Circulation* **106**: 653–8.

Heberden W (1772) Some account of a disorder of the breast. *Medical Transcripts of the College of Physicians* **2**: 59.

Hill R, Bagust A, Bakhai A et al. (2004) Coronary artery stents: a rapid systematic review and economic evaluation. *Health Technology Assessment* **8**: iii–iv, 1–242.

Hjemdahl P, Eriksson S, Held C et al. (2005) Favourable long-term prognosis in stable angina pectoris; an extended follow up of the angina prognosis study in Stockholm (APSIS) *Heart* (online publication as 10.1136/hrt.2004.057703).

IONA Study Group (2005) Determinants of coronary events in patients with stable angina: results from the Impact of Nicorandil in Angina study. *American Heart Journal* **150**: 689.e1–9.

Jain D, Fluck D, Sayer JW (1997) One-stop chest pain clinic can identify high cardiac risk. *Journal of the Royal College of Physicians of London* **31**: 401–4.

Juul-Moller S, Edvasron N, Jahnmatz B et al. (1992) Double blind trial of aspirin in primary prevention of myocardial infarction in patients with stable chronic angina pectoris. SAPAT (Swedish Angina Pectoris Aspirin Trial). *Lancet* **340**: 1421–5.

Lewin R (1999) Improving quality of life in patients with angina. *Heart* **82**: 654–5.

Lewin R, Furze G, Robinson J et al. (2002) A randomised controlled trial of a self-management plan for patients with newly diagnosed angina. *British Journal of General Practice* **52**: 194–201.

McMahan C, Gidding S, Fayad S et al. (2005) Risk scores predict atherosclerotic lesions in young people. *Archives of Internal Medicine* **165**: 883–9.

Mayou R, Bryant B, Forfar C et al. (1994) Non-cardiac chest pain and benign palpitations in the cardiac clinic. *British Heart Journal* 72: 548–553.

National Assembly for Wales (2001) *Tackling CHD in Wales: Implementing through evidence.* Cardiff: Welsh Assembly Government.

Newby D, Fox K, Flint L et al. (1998) A 'same day' direct access chest pain clinic: improved management and reduced hospitalisation. *Quarterly Journal of Medicine* **91**: 333–7.

Nissen S, Tuzcu E, Schoenhagen P et al. (2004) Effect of intensive compared with moderate lipid-lowering therapy on progression of coronary atherosclerosis: a randomized controlled trial. *Journal of the American Medical Association* **291**: 1071–80.

Norell M, Lythall D, Coghlan G et al. (1992) Limited value of the resting electrocardiogram in assessing patients with recent onset chest pain: lessons from a chest pain clinic. *British Heart Journal* **67**: 53–6.

Philpott S, Boynton P, Feder G et al. (2001) Gender differences in descriptions of angina symptoms and health problems immediately prior to angiography: the ACRE study. *Social Science and Medicine* **52**: 1565–75.

Price J, Mayou R, Bass C et al. (2005) Developing a rapid access chest pain clinic: qualitative studies of patients' needs and experiences. *Journal of Psychosomatic Research* **59**: 237–46.

Quinn T, Webster RA, Hatchett R (2002) Coronary heart disease: angina and acute myocardial infarction. In: Hatchett R, Thompson DR (eds), *Cardiac Nursing: A comprehensive guide*. Edinburgh: Churchill Livingstone, pp. 151–188.

Rodgers G, Ayanian J, Balady G et al. (2000) American College of Cardiology/American Heart Association clinical competence statement on stress testing. A report of the American College of Cardiology/American Heart Association/American College of Physicians –American Society of Internal Medicine task force on clinical competence. *Circulation* **102**: 1726–38.

Ross R (1999) Atherosclerosis: an inflammatory disease. *New England Journal of Medicine* **340**: 115–226.

Sangareddi V, Chockalingam A, Gnanavelu G et al. (2004) Canadian Cardiovascular Society classification of effort angina: an angiographic correlation. *Coronary Artery Disease* **15**: 111–14.

Schoenhagen P, Ziada R, Kapadia S et al. (2000) Extent and direction of arterial remodelling in stable versus unstable coronary syndromes: an intravascular ultrasound study. *Circulation* **101**: 598–603.

Scottish Executive Health Department (2002) *Coronary Heart Disease and Stroke Strategy for Scotland.* Edinburgh: The Stationery Office.

Snow V, Barry P, Fihn S et al. (2004) Evaluation of primary care patients with chronic stable angina: guidelines from the American College of Physicians. *Annals of Internal Medicine* **141**: 57–64.

Stewart S, Murphy N, Walker A et al. (2003) The current cost of angina pectoris to the National Health Service in the UK. *Heart* **89**: 848–53.

Sutcliffe S, Fox K, Wood D et al. (2003) Incidence of angina, myocardial infarction and sudden cardiac death – a community register. *British Medical Journal* **326**: 20.

Terkelsen C, Vach W (2005) Commentary: can risk score models help in reducing serious outcome events in patients with stable angina? *British Medical Journal* **331**: 872.

Thompson D, Webster R (2005) *Caring for the Coronary Patient*, 2nd edn. Edinburgh: Elsevier Science.

7 Coronary heart disease: acute coronary syndromes

TOM QUINN

There are an estimated 268 000 episodes of acute myocardial infarction (AMI) in the UK each year (British Heart Foundation or BHF 2004). In England and Wales there are an estimated 700 000 attendances at hospital emergency and accident (A&E) departments because of acute chest pain and associated symptoms (Goodacre et al. 2005). The burden on patients, the NHS and society from acute coronary syndromes (ACS) – whether confirmed or suspected – is therefore substantial.

As described in Chapter 1, death rates from coronary heart disease (CHD) have been falling over recent decades, mostly because of reductions in important risk factors, especially smoking. About 40% of the fall in CHD deaths in England and Wales in recent years has resulted from advances in clinical care (Unal et al. 2004). In patients with ACS, treatment – defibrillation, aspirin, thrombolytic treatment and secondary prevention medication – has made an important contribution (Unal et al. 2004). Further advances in emergency cardiac care, such as very early – increasingly pre-hospital – administration of thrombolytic treatment, and increased availability of percutaneous coronary intervention (PCI) for ACS patients are expected to improve outcomes further.

Although much of the following focuses on immediate care of the patient with a suspected ACS and in particular on 'barn door' ST elevation myocardial infarction, effectiveness of initial treatments and being time dependent, patients with other presentations are at risk of death or other adverse events in the ensuing months and should always be taken seriously. The high incidence of 'undifferentiated chest pain' (Goodacre et al. 2005) has led to the evaluation of strategies such as chest pain observation units that are outside the scope of this book.

Cardiac Care: An Introduction for Healthcare Professionals. Edited by David Barrett, Mark Gretton and Tom Quinn
© 2006 John Wiley & Sons Ltd

DEFINITIONS

Acute coronary syndromes – the clinical syndromes encompassing unstable angina and evolving myocardial infarction (MI) – are a major healthcare problem and result in a large number of hospital admissions each year. In recent years, management of patients with ACS has improved as understanding of the pathological processes behind the condition has grown. The spectrum of ACS conditions can be subdivided on the basis of clinical, ECG and biomarker release findings:

- ST elevation MI (STEMI): symptoms suggestive of acute myocardial ischaemia with persistent ST-segment elevation on the 12-lead ECG, with release of markers of myocardial necrosis.
- Non-ST elevation MI (NSTEMI): symptoms suggestive of acute myocardial ischaemia without persistent ST-segment elevation on the 12-lead ECG (but typically with ST-segment depression or T-wave inversion, or transient ST elevation), with release of markers of myocardial necrosis.
- Unstable angina (UA): symptoms suggestive of acute myocardial ischaemia without persistent ST-segment elevation on the 12-lead ECG (but typically with ST-segment depression or T-wave inversion, or transient ST elevation), and without release of markers of myocardial necrosis.

All manifestations of ACS carry substantial mortality risk but treatment options vary according to ECG presentation, indicating the underlying pathophysiology. Thrombolytic treatment saves lives in patients with persistent ST-segment elevation or left bundle-branch block (LBBB) but appears to worsen outcomes in patients with isolated ST-segment depression (Fibrinolytic Treatment Trialists' Collaborative Group 1994); therefore NSTEMI patients are not given this treatment.

Guidelines for the assessment, risk stratification and treatment of patients with ACS have been published by the American College of Cardiology and the American Heart Association (Antman et al. 2004), and the European Society of Cardiology (Bertrand et al. 2002, Van de Werf et al. 2003). In England, the National Service Framework (NSF) for CHD (Department of Health or DH 2000) set national standards for improved prevention and treatment. Other British countries have set similar standards for cardiac care (National Assembly for Wales 2001, Scottish Executive 2002).

THE CARDIAC CARE UNIT

Acute cardiac care has evolved markedly from the time of the first coronary (or cardiac) care units (CCUs), developed in the 1960s to reduce deaths from arrhythmia. CCUs provided a specialised facility to monitor patients with suspected MI and to facilitate rapid defibrillation of patients in cardiac arrest

(Julian 1987). Nurses trained in resuscitation were crucial to the provision of 24-hour expertise in rhythm recognition and early defibrillation to patients at the bedside. The CCU has survived as a service in most acute hospitals in spite of early controversy about the effectiveness of this model when compared with home care (Rawles and Kenmure 1980).

The success of the CCU concept is highly reliant on multidisciplinary effort. CCU nurses and doctors together pioneered the specialist knowledge and skill in electrocardiogram (ECG) interpretation and treatment of adverse events, including cardiopulmonary resuscitation (CPR), which was seen previously as the sole preserve of the physician (Meltzer 1964). The development of the CCU arguably provides the earliest examples of nurses taking on 'enhanced' roles (Killip and Kimball 1967). Recommendations for the structure, organisation and operation of 'intensive cardiac care units' have been published by the European Society of Cardiology working group on acute cardiac care (Hasin et al. 2005) and, for the first time in a document of this type, recommendations for nurse staffing levels have been made. Recent years have seen marked devolution of cardiac care to A&E and ambulance clinicians (Quinn et al. 2002, Quinn and Morse 2003) such that the role of the CCU is being reappraised (Quinn et al. 2005b).

REPERFUSION TREATMENTS IN STEMI

The introduction of intravenous thrombolytic treatment into routine management of MI came after the publication of large trials in the mid-1980s, followed by a range of policy and professional initiatives to increase uptake and speed of care (Cook et al. 2004). Clinical trials provided strong evidence that the sooner suitable patients with MI were treated with a thrombolytic agent the better their chances of survival (Fibrinolytic Therapy Trialists' Collaborative Group 1994). A meta-analysis of both hospital and pre-hospital thrombolysis trials has reinforced the time-dependent nature of this treatment (Boersma et al. 1996): the concept of a 'golden hour' for thrombolysis has been proposed (Boersma al 1996), although this may underestimate the benefits (Terkelsen et al. 2004). The importance of very early treatment has been reinforced by recent studies comparing thrombolytic treatment with primary percutaneous coronary intervention (PPCI), which is discussed later.

For patients with symptoms suggesting a heart attack who present with STEMI or new left bundle-branch block (LBBB) on the 12-lead ECG, the NSF standards relate to reducing delay so that patients begin thrombolytic treatment within 60 minutes of the call for professional help. An early focus on optimising hospital systems so that patients started thrombolysis within 20–30 minutes of arrival subsequently shifted to starting treatment within 60 minutes 'call-to-needle time' (Department of Health 2003). The national audit of MI (MINAP) for England and Wales has reported more than three-quarters of eligible MI patients starting thrombolysis within 30 minutes of hospital arrival (Birkhead et al. 2004), a major factor being the shift from CCU to A&E as the main place where thrombolysis is given. Thrombolysis in A&E is feasible and safe, and adverse incidents including cardiac arrest during subsequent transfer to CCU are rare (Edhouse et al. 1999). Before publication of the NSF, few A&E departments were providing this treatment (Hood et al. 1998). Direct CCU admission has largely been superseded by A&E care although it is possible that direct admission to a cardiac catheter laboratory for PCI may become more widely available in future.

Half of all eligible patients receive immediate thrombolytic treatment within 60 minutes of calling for help (MINAP 2005). Further reductions in delay will depend on wider use of pre-hospital thrombolysis, delivered mostly by paramedics (Boyle 2004). Pre-hospital thrombolysis has been the subject of a meta-analysis, which demonstrated a 17% reduction in all-cause mortality (Morrison et al. 2000) compared with hospital thrombolysis. Keeling et al. (2003) reported that autonomous paramedic administration of thrombolysis was feasible and safe and improved call-to-needle times. Pedley et al. (2003) demonstrated that the proportion of STEMI patients starting treatment within 60 minutes of the call was markedly improved when pre-hospital thrombolysis was available. Several thousand patients in England have received thrombolysis from a paramedic since the publication of the NSF (Ambulance Service Association 2005). The balance between risk and benefit of providing pre-hospital thrombolysis in an urban setting, with presumed short transport times, has been subject to debate (Stephenson et al. 2002) and the precise model adopted (increasingly including PCI) depends on local circumstances.

PATIENT CARE – PRIORITIES AND PATHWAYS

The care of the patient with symptoms suggestive of an ACS requires a combination of clinical assessment skill and knowledge, compassion and communication, and speed. Patients and family members may be highly anxious and distressed and the clinician needs to approach the situation in a calm and reassuring manner. Patients with ACS and other manifestations of CHD value being treated with respect by competent practitioners – and they also rate adequate pain relief and information giving as priorities (Quinn et al. 2005a). The high incidence of CHD in some minority ethnic populations may present additional cultural and language considerations that require sensitivity alongside an appreciation that treatment delays are longer, and outcomes worse, in this group. People with learning difficulties, and those with mental health problems, are not immune from CHD. The clinician, whose goal is to reduce the risk of death and disability for the patient, must consider all these issues.

As the benefits of main treatments for STEMI patients are time related, the clinician must work with the patient rapidly to obtain a working diagnosis and initiate appropriate treatment. This section focuses on this early phase of care. As early priorities are similar whatever the ECG manifestation, the following should provide a guide for patient assessment and care whether or not there is ECG evidence of STEMI.

The key steps in the ACS patient pathway have been described in terms of the '4Ds' denoting door, data, decision and drug (National Heart Attack Alert Program 1994). These have been adapted for use in the British setting by Quinn and Thompson (1995) and can now be updated for contemporary practice:

- D0 – domicile: patient, family member or bystander recognition of symptoms of 'heart attack' and consequent help-seeking behaviour.
- D1 – door: initial assessment, resuscitation and triage by first healthcare contact, whether ambulance clinician or first responder (or hospital staff if the patient self-presents).
- D2 – data: rapid history taking and focused clinical assessment, including acquisition and interpretation of the first 12-lead ECG.
- D3 – decision: use of the data from D2 to form a working diagnosis and determine eligibility for reperfusion treatment as the key time-dependent priority.
- D4 – drug or destination: once eligibility for reperfusion treatment has been established, administration of a thrombolytic should begin immediately and the patient transferred to an appropriate hospital. Alternatively, the STEMI patient should be transferred as an emergency to the nearest interventional centre. The destination of the patient without evidence of STEMI will depend on local policy.

D0 – DOMICILE

This stage relates patient recognition of symptoms of 'heart attack' and help-seeking behaviour.

Although 'call-to-needle' times for thrombolysis in STEMI patients have improved over recent years, patients are taking longer to call for help after symptom onset (Birkhead et al. 2004) and thus overall delay from symptom onset to starting treatment – a major determinant of outcome – may increase. Help-seeking behaviour determines the speed of availability not only of reperfusion, but also of a defibrillator – defibrillation potentially saves more lives than reperfusion strategies (Julian and Norris 2002) – and the prognosis of patients successfully resuscitated from early ventricular fibrillation (VF) is the same as that of patients who have not had VF (Sayer et al. 2000). A recent systematic review concluded that there was little evidence that media or public education interventions reduced delay, and that there is some evidence that they may result in an increase in emergency switchboard calls and A&E visits which may place an additional burden on such services (Kainth et al. 2004). There is no 'magic message' proven consistently to improve patient delay.

D1 – DOOR

As the risk of death from arrhythmia is high in the early hours from symptom onset in ACS patients, the first priority is to ensure the rapid availability of a defibrillator, and someone who can use it, at the patient's side. The evidence that survival rates from cardiac arrest are highest when an arrest is witnessed by an ambulance crew (Norris 1998), and that the likelihood of successful resuscitation from cardiac arrest diminishes rapidly over a few minutes, has resulted in standards of care mandating rapid ambulance response times (DH 2000) and the use of community first responders trained in defibrillation, together with widespread availability of automated defibrillators in public places (Davies et al. 2002). Resuscitation is discussed in more detail in Chapter 10. The defibrillator should remain at the patient's side until handover to competent staff where resuscitation facilities are immediately available in hospital. Many modern devices carried by ambulances and in A&E departments facilitate continuous monitoring of blood pressure and oxygen saturation in addition to ECG.

Initial steps in the assessment process include establishing presence of vital signs and conscious level: the simple 'ABCs' of airway, breathing and circulation apply to the emergency cardiac patient as to any other. On establishing that the patient does not require immediate resuscitation, a rapid, focused assessment is required to identify the chief complaint (why the patient sought help), identify any risk factors for deterioration that might require immediate attention (e.g. profound bradycardia and hypotension, or signs of acute heart failure), measure and manage pain, and establish a working diagnosis. Many patients will not have a final diagnosis of ACS (Goodacre et al. 2005). Key areas for attention in the emergency setting are discussed below.

D2 – DATA

This involves rapid history taking and focused clinical assessment, including acquisition and interpretation of the first 12-lead ECG. Establishing the time and duration of symptom onset, if known, is important because of the time-related benefits of treatments such as thrombolysis. It is important to note whether any chest pain or discomfort was of gradual or sudden onset because more sudden onset might indicate aortic dissection rather than ACS as a cause, requiring immediate transfer to a suitable hospital for further specialist assessment. Symptom characteristics (e.g. constricting, radiating or stabbing pain) and any precipitating or aggravating factors (e.g. recent trauma, pain worse on inspiration or improved by position change) may help to distinguish ACS from more benign causes. Associated symptoms (e.g. nausea, sweating), whether symptoms are new or recurrent, if the patient has a past history of 'heart attack' or angina, and whether the current episode is of a similar nature to previous symptoms can all help the clinician to form an initial clinical judgement about whether the patient is suffering 'cardiac' pain. Assessment of ischaemic pain is explored in more detail in Chapter 5.

Initial management at this stage should also include administration of supplemental oxygen and aspirin – which saves as many lives as streptokinase alone (ISIS-2 [Second International Study of Infarct Survival] 1988) – and should be given promptly unless an absolute contraindication exists), and nitrate spray or sublingual tablet should be given for ongoing chest discomfort. Opiate analgesia may be required for severe symptoms and will require intravenous access – the increased mortality seen in ACS patients given morphine in one observational study (Meine et al. 2005) was probably a result of sicker patients receiving morphine: opiate analgesia should not be denied to patients in pain. Rhythm abnormalities causing symptoms or associated with other adverse signs may require immediate treatment.

Clinical impressions alone are an insufficient basis on which to make treatment decisions in the context of a suspected ACS. As discussed above, different manifestations of ACS require different treatments: STEMI patients may benefit from thrombolytic treatment whereas those with NSTEMI will not. It is important therefore to obtain a 12-lead ECG recording at the earliest opportunity. The aim should be for a first ECG to be recorded within 5–10 minutes of first contact with the patient. All emergency ambulances in England are equipped with 12-lead ECG machines. The requirement for a very early ECG recording applies in hospital if patients self-present or have not had an ECG recorded by ambulance staff. The use of aspirin administration as a 'trigger' to record a 12-lead ECG in the setting of a suspected ACS has been recommended (Woollard and Quinn 2005).

Very early ECG recordings by ambulance clinicians

Recording and interpreting the 12-lead ECG are discussed in Chapter 5. Many ambulance services collaborate with local hospitals within clinical networks to facilitate transmission of ECGs for interpretation or advice from hospital clinicians. There is evidence that suitably trained paramedics can accurately identify STEMI for the purposes of recommending thrombolysis (Whitbread et al. 2002), skills that could arguably be utilised to refer patients for primary PCI without the need first to take the patient to a non-interventional centre (Quinn and Whitbread 2005).

In the pre-hospital setting it may be appropriate to record the ECG and continue the patient assessment and management in the ambulance while en route to hospital to reduce delay, although it can also be argued that most of the initial assessment and care could reasonably take place indoors before moving the patient to the ambulance: the precise actions will depend on the judgement of the attending paramedic or other clinician. Transmission of the 12-lead ECG in a moving ambulance has been shown to be feasible and safe (Giovas et al. 1998, Papouchado et al. 2001). Although studies have tended to be small, meta-analyses have confirmed the usefulness of the ECG in the pre-hospital setting. (Ioannidis et al. 2001, Brainard et al. 2005). In one study cardiologists made similar treatment decisions regarding thrombolysis when they received an ECG transmitted by telemetry to a mobile phone 'communicator' as when they were faced with a conventional printed ECG (Leibrandt et al. 2000): this technology is now used extensively within Staffordshire Ambulance Service in England, facilitating by far the largest number of patients receiving pre-hospital thrombolysis in a British ambulance setting (Quinn et al. 2006). One recent randomised trial of ambulance ECG telemetry suggested that the benefits of such a system were limited by junior doctors' reluctance to make treatment decisions remotely on patients and that technical difficulties meant that ECG transmission was unreliable (Woollard et al. 2005). These findings highlight the importance of carefully selecting equipment and processes appropriate to the setting and task in hand, and involving all relevant personnel in developing operating procedures for changes in practice. Clinical governance issues arising from ECG transmission have been highlighted by Quinn et al. (2002).

Biomarkers

Although the use of biomarkers (e.g. troponin, myoglobin) to identify and support risk stratification in patients with ACS is standard practice in the hospital setting, their use in the ambulance setting has thus far been studied solely on the basis of assessing the feasibility of performing the test out of hospital and in evaluating their performance in predicting short- and long-term risk of death (Svennson et al. 2004). There is no evidence that biomarker-positive patients who do not have STEMI benefit from reperfusion treatment. Moreover, the causes of raised troponins extend beyond ACS to include at least 25 other conditions identified by Ammann et al. (2005), ranging from cardiac amyloidosis to ultra-endurance (marathon running) exercise. Any test should be interpreted in the context of the whole clinical assessment of the patient.

D3 – DECISION

The key decision required in the early stages of care of the patient with a suspected ACS relates to eligibility for reperfusion treatment, whether pharmacological (thrombolysis) or mechanical (PCI). This decision is based on a combination of clinical assessment and the 12-lead ECG as discussed above.

In determining the initial treatment strategy, the clinician is required to balance the risks and benefits of treatment. Patients with STEMI require urgent treatment to reduce mortality as a top priority, but the benefits of thrombolytic treatment need to be weighed against the risk of increased bleeding risk, in particular intracranial haemorrhage, e.g. a patient with STEMI who has severe hypertension, is of low body weight and advanced age (>75–80 years of age) might be better served by being transferred for PCI than by being given thrombolysis. Patients with STEMI who have contraindications to thrombolytic treatment or are otherwise ineligible tend to have worse outcomes and would also benefit from transfer for emergency angiography and possible PCI. In some settings PCI is being provided as routine for all STEMI patients in preference to thrombolysis. Guidelines and checklists agreed locally are useful in helping clinicians to make these judgements.

A small proportion (about 6%) of MI patients will present with LBBB on the ECG. In the presence of MI, LBBB carries a very high mortality – in over 600 patients with MI studied by Terkelsen et al. (2005), 55% of patients with LBBB died within a year, compared with 21% of STEMI and 31% of NSTEMI patients. As many patients who have LBBB are not having an MI, however, decision-making on emergency treatment can be difficult and senior advice is recommended. Decision-making must be rapid because treatment delays in the setting of a STEMI can adversely influence the outcome for the patient. This is important for patients receiving thrombolysis, where an estimated 11 days of life are lost for every minute's delay (Rawles 1997). For PCI the mortality risk increased by 7.5% for every 30 minutes of additional delay in initiating treatment (De Luca et al. 2004).

Most patients with acute chest pain will not have an ACS diagnosis, and a minority of those with ACSs will have STEMI and require immediate reperfusion. The specific management of NSTEMI and unstable angina ACS patients is discussed later.

D4 – WHICH DRUG (IF ANY)? WHICH DESTINATION?

Once the decision has been made that a patient does, or does not, require reperfusion treatment, the priorities switch to delivering the treatment, or getting the patient safely to an appropriate hospital or department for further assessment and care. A growing number of patients are receiving thrombolytic treatment from ambulance staff. Government and professions alike have acknowledged the key role of paramedics and other clinicians in expediting treatment through better collaboration between hospitals and emergency services. At the time of writing, the majority of thrombolysis is administered in hospital A&E departments but this is predicted to change: in the next few years more patients with STEMI will either receive pre-hospital thrombolysis or, where facilities exist, be transferred to specialist MI centres (Andersen et al. 2005, Bassand et al. 2005, Quinn and Whitbread 2005). Some health systems have already introduced networks of 'STEMI' and 'NSTEMI' hospitals, whereby patients who require immediate reperfusion bypass local general hospitals for tertiary centres; local general hospitals in such systems retain responsibility for the care of patients with other manifestations of ACS that are less time dependent (Moyer et al. 2004).

The choice of thrombolytic drug, if indicated, will be dictated by local policies. Although much has been made of findings from one trial (GUSTO 1993) suggesting apparent benefit of alteplase over streptokinase, a review of the comparative clinical effectiveness of newer thrombolytic agents (reteplase and tenecteplase) with older agents (alteplase and streptokinase) concluded that all appear to be of similar efficacy in reducing mortality (Dundar et al. 2003). The newer agents, which are administered as bolus injections, have been recommended for pre-hospital administration based on their ease of use; streptokinase continues to be recommended for use in hospital in patients with their first MI (National Institute for Clinical Excellence or NICE 2002). Moreover, Heyland et al. (2000) reported that, when provided with data on the relative merits and risks of alteplase and streptokinase, over half of non-MI patients with CHD (and therefore potential recipients of thrombolysis in the future) indicated a preference for streptokinase on the basis of a potentially lower risk of stroke. These considerations need to be balanced against suboptimal restoration of coronary blood flow in patients treated with streptokinase (30%) compared with alteplase (54%) or reteplase (56%) (Stringer 1998). PCI has been reported to restore near-normal coronary blood flow in more than 90% of patients (Grines et al. 1993). Both currently available 'bolus' thrombolytic agents require adjunctive heparin and clinical trials are ongoing to determine the optimal regimen. The issues are complex: the mortality and coronary artery patency benefits of low-molecular-weight heparin (LMWH), in comparison with unfractionated heparin, have to be balanced against increased intracranial haemorrhage in older patients (Brouwer et al. 2004).

The benefits of aspirin in reducing mortality from AMI are about equal to those of streptokinase alone (ISIS-2 1998). Another medicine gaining widespread acceptance in the care of the patient with ACS is clopidogrel which, when used as an addition to thrombolysis and aspirin, improved patency of the infarct-related coronary artery and reduced ischaemic complications in STEMI patients aged 75 years or younger (Sabatine et al. 2005). Studies of the addition of platelet glycoprotein IIb/IIIa inhibitor agents to thrombolytic treatment have identified a significant additional risk of intracranial haemorrhage in older patients with STEMI (Savonitto et al. 2003). Some authors have recently suggested that administration of a IIb/IIIa inhibitor, eptifibatide, in the pre-hospital setting on clinical suspicion of ACS (including STEMI) is feasible and safe. (Hanefeld et al. 2004) More studies in this area of care are under way. Cardiac medications are discussed in more detail in Chapter 13.

Mechanical reperfusion

The superiority of primary PCI over hospital-delivered thrombolytic treatment has been demonstrated conclusively by a meta-analysis of 23 randomised trials (Keeley et al. 2003). The combined endpoint of death, non-fatal reinfarction and stroke was 8% in PCI patients versus 14% in those who received thrombolysis. This study has been very influential in stimulating debate across the health service in England about how best to provide care for patients with MI. There is not, however, unanimity concerning wholesale change in service provision for MI patients. Patients randomised to PCI trials may not have been representative of 'usual practice' and may have been at lower baseline risk of death compared with thrombolysis patients, and there are methodological concerns about some of the trials reported (de Jaegere et al. 2004). Availability of a PCI service on a 24-hour, 7-day-a-week basis and sufficient volume of activity to ensure technical expertise are additional considerations, which are being tested in a feasibility study funded by the Department of Health in England (DH 2004).

There is insufficient evidence to recommend that every patient with acute MI should be transferred for primary PCI (de Jaegere et al. 2004), although this is a subject of controversy (Keeley et al. 2004) and international guidelines suggest that, where promptly available, PCI is the preferred option (Van de Werf et al. 2003, Antman et al. 2004). Other authorities suggest that both treatments are reasonable options for patients with MI (Brophy and Bogaty 2004), or that a strategy of facilitated PCI following pre-hospital thrombolytic administration may be preferable (Schofield 2005, Townend and Doshi 2005). The European Society of Cardiology recommend PCI if it can be performed by experienced staff within 90 minutes of initial medical contact and, alternatively, thrombolytic treatment – pre-hospital where possible – if PCI is not immediately available, and especially in patients presenting within 3 hours of symptom onset where the mortality advantage of PCI over thrombolysis is not as well established (Bassand et al. 2005).

ONGOING CARDIAC CARE AND ASSESSMENT

The care of the patient with suspected ACS does not end when the immediate assessment and treatment phase has been accomplished. Patients undergoing thrombolytic treatment require ongoing monitoring of ECG and other vital signs. The clinician must be ready to manage significant arrhythmias immediately; although the risk of primary VF is the same whether or not thrombolysis is given, the incidence of later or 'secondary' VF may be higher in patients who do not get reperfusion treatment (Solomon et al. 1993). Recurrent or unresolved pain and breathlessness, high or low blood pressure and arrhythmias giving rise to adverse signs require urgent remedy. The availability of a 12-lead ECG 90 minutes after initiation of reperfusion treatment allows measurement of ST-segment resolution that can provide useful prognostic information. Those patients in whom thrombolytic treatment has 'failed' (i.e. symptoms and ST-segment elevation persist), in whom recurrent symptoms and new ST elevation suggest reocclusion of the infarct-related coronary artery or reinfarction, or who develop shock, should be assessed promptly for rescue PCI (Van de Werf et al. 2003, Gershlick et al. 2005).

RISK STRATIFICATION IN THE ACS PATIENT WITHOUT STEMI

The burden of NSTEMI ACS on patients and health services is considerable. Although hospital admission rates for MI are reportedly falling, there has been a marked increase in hospitalisations for other ACS in recent years with potentially enormous implications for resources, including a need for expansion of interventional facilities (Murphy et al. 2004). For patients presenting without persistent ST-segment elevation, early risk stratification plays a central role because benefits of a more aggressive treatment regimen appear to be proportional to the risk of complications (Goncalves et al. 2005). Whereas decisions about reperfusion treatments are based largely on the initial ECG (STEMI or BBB required), further characterisation of NSTEMI or unstable angina manifestations of ACS require measurement of biochemical markers to detect myocardial necrosis, as discussed above.

Initial treatment of the NSTEMI or unstable angina patient is based on medical management with aspirin, clopidogrel and LMWH. Persistent or recurrent chest pain usually requires treatment with β blockers and oral or intravenous nitrates. Where contraindications exist, clopidogrel can be used in place of aspirin, and calcium channel blockers can replace β blockers (see Chapter 13).

Patients must be closely observed for recurrent pain (a 12-lead ECG should be recorded as a matter of urgency – continuous ST-segment monitoring may be useful if available), and signs of haemodynamic instability such as breathlessness, hypotension or arrhythmia require urgent senior advice. Patients require close monitoring; although many patients with NSTEMI or unstable angina are managed on general medical wards, this is considered suboptimal care (Quinn et al. 2005b).

Risk stratification is accomplished using information gained from clinical, ECG and biochemical tests. A number of risk 'scores' have been developed to assist with this process by providing objective measurements of risk derived from clinical trials. The commonly used scores provide information on short-term risk as shown in Table 7.1.

When performance of these three scores was compared by Goncalves et al. (2005), each demonstrated good predictive accuracy for death or MI at 1 year

Table 7.1 Summary of principal elements of three acute coronary syndrome risk scores

Risk score	Key criteria	Predicts risk of events at *n* days
TIMI (Antman et al. 2000)	Age, CHD risk factors, aspirin use, known CHD, ST-segment deviation, cardiac marker release	14 days
PURSUIT (Boersma et al. 2000)	Age, sex, angina score, heart failure and ST depression	30 days
GRACE (Granger et al. 2003)	Age, heart rate, systolic BP, creatinine, Killip class, cardiac arrest, elevated markers, ST-segment deviation	In hospital events, 6-month event rate

From Goncalves et al. (2005).

Table 7.2 Risk characteristics of ACS patients

High-risk characteristics	Low-risk characteristics
Recurrent ischaemia	No recurrence of chest pain during observation period
Recurrent chest pain	No marker (e.g. troponin) elevation[a]
Dynamic ST-segment changes	No ST-segment deviation
Early post-MI unstable angina	Negative or flat T waves
Elevated troponin levels	Normal ECG
Diabetes	
Haemodynamic instability	
Major arrhythmias (VF, VT)	

[a]Including second negative troponin at 6–12 hours.
ACS, acute coronary syndrome; MI, myocardial infarction; VF, ventricular fibrillation; VT, ventricular tachycardia.
Adapted from Bertrand et al. (2002).

from the initial ACS admission, enabling decisions to be made about which patients would benefit most from invasive management (myocardial revascularisation using PCI or CAB grafts) during hospitalisation. Whichever risk score is used locally, ACS patients can generally be divided into 'high' and 'low' risk for the purposes of decision-making, with regard to the use of more aggressive treatments. The European Society of Cardiology has summarised the key characteristics of these groups as shown in Table 7.2.

Patients considered at high risk require angiography (see Chapter 14) as soon as practicable, although this is not generally as time dependent as for patients with STEMI who are undergoing PCI. Patients should, however, remain in hospital under observation while awaiting the procedure. This can cause logistical challenges where a hospital does not have on-site interventional facilities (Miller et al. 2003).

Patients categorised as 'low risk' should continue on medical management (although heparin can be discontinued once the second troponin measurement is negative). An exercise tolerance test should be performed before discharge from hospital.

ANXIETY IN PATIENTS AND RELATIVES

There is little doubt that hospitalisation with a 'heart attack', whether STEMI or NSTEMI, will be a time of considerable anxiety for patients and their loved ones, conjuring up images of premature death, disability, and the possibility of changes in employment, family roles and relationships (Quinn 1998). Exposure to the high-technology world of the ambulance, A&E and CCU will be anxiety provoking; equipment – not least the bleeps and alarms that characterise the critical care environment – will be unfamiliar and may serve only to confirm the presence of serious illness and possibility of death. Patients and loved ones will require information and reassurance. As most patients are conscious throughout their heart attack 'journey', rehabilitation should ideally begin as soon as possible, while avoiding information overload.

The needs of relatives are important and can be unrecognised, and are not universally well met. Emotional and physical distress, with feelings of helplessness, disorganisation and difficulty in coping, are common. Anxiety, depression, guilt, sleep disturbance and fatigue may be experienced (O'Malley et al. 1991). Key stressors include inability to discuss progress with a doctor, long travelling distances to visit, restricted visiting hours and uncomfortable waiting conditions. Not knowing whom to turn to for advice and information is another cause of stress.

MAKING THE TRANSITION FROM CCU TO THE GENERAL WARD

Much early rehabilitation will take place on a lower dependency ward as – bed state and clinical condition permitting – the stay on CCU is often less than 1 or 2 days. Patients often experience anxiety about moving from what they perceive as the 'safe haven' of a comparatively well-staffed CCU to a ward where monitoring may be less intense. Cardiac rehabilitation is discussed in more depth in Chapter 3.

CONCLUSION

Major advances in the medical treatment of patients with AMI and other manifestations of ACS have been introduced into routine practice over the past two decades, saving many thousands of lives. Experience is growing in the prehospital management of patients with STEMI presentations in particular, and our understanding of the pathophysiology of other manifestations of ACSs is now being translated into changes in clinical practice and improved outcomes. The large number of patients with acute chest pain in whom an ACS diagnosis is not immediately apparent presents a significant challenge for healthcare professionals in the future.

REFERENCES

Ambulance Service Association (2005) *Thrombolysis update*: www.asancep.org.uk (accessed 9 July 2005).

Ammann P, Pfisterer M, Fehr T et al. (2005) Raised cardiac troponins. *British Medical Journal* **328**: 1028–9.

Andersen H, Terkelsen C, Thuesen L et al. (2005) Myocardial infarction centres: the way forward. *Heart* **91**(suppl III): 12–15.

Antman EM, Cohen M, Bernink PJ et al. (2000) The TIMI risk score for unstable angina/non-ST elevation MI. *Journal of the American Medical Association* **284**: 835–42.

Antman E, Anbe D, Armstrong P et al. (2004) ACC/AHA guidelines for the management of patients with ST-elevation myocardial infarction. A report of the American College of Cardiology/American Heart Association Task Force on Practice Guidelines (Committee to Revise the 1999 Guidelines for the Management of patients with acute myocardial infarction). *Journal of the American College of Cardiology* 44: E1–211.

Bassand JP, Danchin N, Filippatos G et al. (2005) Implementation of reperfusion therapy in acute myocardial infarction. A policy statement from the European Society of Cardiology. *European Heart Journal* **26**: 2733–41.

Bertrand M, Simoons ML, Fox K et al. (2002) Management of acute coronary syndromes in patients presenting without persistent ST segment elevation. Task Force of the ESC. *European Heart Journal* **23**: 1809–40.

Birkhead J, Walker L, Pearson M et al. (2004) Improving care for patients with acute coronary syndromes: initial results from the National Audit of Myocardial Infarction Project (MINAP) *Heart* **90**: 1004–9.

Boersma E, Maas C, Deckers J et al. (1996) Early thrombolytic treatment in acute myocardial infarction: reappraisal of the golden hour. *Lancet* **348**: 771–5.

Boersma E, Pieper KS, Steyerberg EW et al. for the PURSUIT Investigators (2000) Predictors of outcome in patients with acute coronary syndromes without persistent ST-segment elevation. Results from an international trial of 9461 patients. *Circulation* **101**: 2557–67.

Boyle R (2004) *MINAP Third Public Report*. Dear Colleague letter. Available from www.dh.gov.uk/assetRoot/04/08/40/28/04084028.pdf

Brainard A, Raynovich W, Tandberg D et al. (2005) The prehospital 12 lead electrocardiogram's effect on time to initiation of reperfusion therapy: a systematic review and meta-analysis of existing literature. *American Journal of Emergency Medicine* **23**: 351–6.

British Heart Foundation (2004) *Coronary Heart Disease Statistics Database*: www.heartstats.org

Brophy J, Bogaty P (2004) Primary angioplasty and thrombolysis are both reasonable options in acute myocardial infarction. *Annals of Internal Medicine* **141**: 292–7.

Brouwer M, Clappers N, Verheugt F (2004) Adjunctive treatment in patients treated with thrombolytic therapy. *Heart* **90**: 581–8.

Cook A, Packer C, Stevens A et al. (2004) Influences upon the diffusion of thrombolysis for acute myocardial infarction in England: case study. *International Journal of Technology Assessment in Health Care* **20**: 537–44.

Davies C, Colquhoun M, Graham S et al. (2002) Defibrillators in public places: the introduction of a national scheme for public access defibrillation in England. *Resuscitation* **52**: 13–21.

de Jaegere P, Serryus P, Simoons M (2004) Should all patients with an acute myocardial infarction be transferred for direct PTCA? *Heart* **90**: 1352–7.

De Luca G, Suryapranata H, Ottervanger J et al. (2004) Time delay to treatment and mortality in primary angioplasty for acute myocardial infarction: every minute of delay counts. *Circulation* **109**: 1223–5.

Department of Health (2000) *National Service Framework for Coronary Heart Disease*. London: Department of Health.

Department of Health (2003) *Review of Early Thrombolysis*. London: Department of Health.

Department of Health (2004) *Winning the War on Heart Disease*. London: Department of Health.

Dundar Y, Hill R, Dickson R et al. (2003) Comparative efficacy of thrombolytics in acute myocardial infarction: a systematic review. *Quarterly Journal of Medicine* **96**: 103–13.

Edhouse J, Sakr M, Wardrope J et al. (1999) Thrombolysis in acute myocardial infarction: the safety and efficiency of treatment in the accident and emergency department. *Journal of Accident and Emergency Medicine* **16**: 325–30.

Fibrinolytic Therapy Trialists' Collaborative Group (1994) Indications for fibrinolytic therapy in suspected acute myocardial infarction: collaborative overview of early mortality and major morbidity results from all randomised trials of more than 1000 patients, *Lancet* **343**: 311–22.

Gershlick AH, Stephens-Lloyd A, Hughes S et al. (2005) Rescue angioplasty after failed thrombolytic therapy for acute myocardial infarction. *New England Journal of Medicine* **353**: 2758–68.

Giovas P, Papadoyannis D, Thomakos D (1998) Transmission of electrocardiograms from a moving ambulance. *Journal of Telemedicine and Telecare* **4**(suppl 1): 5–7.

Goncalves P, Ferreira J, Aguiar C et al. (2005) TIMI, PIRSUIT and GRACE risk scores: sustained prognostic value and interaction with revascularisation in NSTE-ACS. *European Heart Journal* **26**: 865–72.

Goodacre S, Cross E, Arnold J et al. (2005) The health care burden of acute chest pain. *Heart* **91**: 229–30.

Granger CB, Goldberg RJ, Dabbous OH et al. for the Global Registry of Acute Coronary Events Investigators (2003) Predictors of hospital mortality in the global registry of acute coronary events. *Archives of Internal Medicine* **163**: 2345–53.

Grines C, Browne K, Marco J et al. (1993) A comparison of immediate angioplasty with thrombolytic therapy for acute myocardial infarction. The Primary Angioplasty in Myocardial Infarction Study Group. *New England Journal of Medicine* **328**: 673–9.

GUSTO (1993) An international randomized trial comparing four thrombolytic strategies for acute myocardial infarction. The GUSTO investigators. *New England Journal of Medicine* **329**: 673–82.

Hanefeld C, Sirtl C, Spiecker M et al. (2004) Prehospital therapy with the platelet IIb/IIa inhibitor eptifibatide in patients with suspected acute coronary syndromes. *Chest* **126**: 935–41.

Hasin Y, Danchin N, Filippatos G et al. on behalf of the working group on acute cardiac care of the European Society of Cardiology (2005) Recommendations for the structure, organization and operation of intensive cardiac care units. *European Heart Journal* **26**: 1676–82.

Heyland D, Gafni A, Levine M (2000) Do potential patients prefer tissue plasminogen activator (TPA) over streptokinase? An evaluation of the risks and benefits of TPA from the patient's perspective. *Journal of Clinical Epidemiology* **53**: 888–94.

Hood S, Birnie D, Swan L et al. (1998) Questionnaire survey of thrombolytic treatment in accident and emergency departments in the United Kingdom. *British Medical Journal* **316**: 274.

Ioannidis J, Salem D, Chew P et al. (2001) Accuracy and clinical effectiveness of prehospital ECG: a meta-analysis. *Annals of Emergency Medicine* **37**: 461–70.

ISIS-2 (Second International Study of Infarct Survival) Collaborative Group (1988) Randomised trial of intravenous streptokinase, oral aspirin, both, or neither among 17,187 cases of suspected acute myocardial infarction: ISIS-2. *Lancet* **ii**: 349–60.

Julian DG (1987) The history of coronary care units. *British Heart Journal* **57**: 497–502.

Julian DG, Norris RM (2002) Myocardial infarction: is evidence-based medicine the best? *Lancet* **359**: 1515–16.

Kainth A, Hewitt A, Sowden A et al. (2004) Systematic review of interventions to reduce delay in patients with suspected heart attack. *Emergency Medicine Journal* **21**: 506–8.

Keeley E, Grines C (2004) Primary percutaneous intervention for every patient with ST segment elevation myocardial infarction: what stands in the way? *Annals of Internal Medicine* **141**: 298–304.

Keeley E, Boura J, Grines C (2003) Primary angioplasty versus intravenous thrombolytic therapy for acute myocardial infarction: a quantitative review of 23 randomised trials. *Lancet* **361**: 13–20.

Keeling P, Hughes D, Price L et al. (2003) Safety and feasibility of prehospital thrombolysis carried out by paramedics *British Medical Journal* **327**: 37–8.

Killip T, Kimball JT (1967) Treatment of myocardial infarction in a coronary care unit. A two-year experience with 250 patients. *American Journal of Cardiology* **20**: 457–64.

Leibrandt P, Bell S, Savona M (2000) Validation of cardiologists' decisions to initiate reperfusion therapy for acute myocardial infarction with electrocardiograms viewed on liquid crystal displays of cellular telephones. *American Heart Journal* 140: 747–752.

Meine T, Roe M, Chen A et al. (2005) Association of intravenous morphine use and outcomes in acute coronary syndromes: results from the CRUSADE quality improvement initiative. *American Heart Journal* **149**: 1043–9.

Meltzer L (1964) The concept and system of intensive coronary care. *Academy of Medicine New Jersey Bulletin* **10**: 304–11.

Miller C, Lipscomb K, Curzen N (2003) Are district hospital patients with unstable angina at a disadvantage? *Postgraduate Medical Journal* **79**: 485.

MINAP (Myocardial Infarction National Audit Project) (2005) How the NHS manages heart attacks Available from www.rcplondon.ac.uk/pubs/books/minap05

Morrison L, Verbeek P, McDonald A et al. (2000) Mortality and pre-hospital thrombolysis for acute myocardial infarction – a meta analysis. *Journal of the American Medical Association* **283**: 2686–92.

Moyer P, Feldman J, Levine J et al. (2004) Implications of the mechanical (PCI) vs thrombolytic controversy for ST segment elevation myocardial infarction on the organisation of emergency medical services. The Boston EMS experience. *Critical Pathways in Cardiology* **3**: 53–61.

Murphy N, MacIntyre K, Capewell S et al. (2004) Hospital discharge rates for suspected acute coronary syndromes between 1990 and 2000: population based analysis. *British Medical Journal* **328**: 1413–14.

National Assembly for Wales (2001) *Tackling CHD in Wales: Implementing through evidence.* Cardiff: Welsh Assembly Government.

National Heart Attack Alert Program (1994) Emergency department: rapid identification and treatment of patients with acute myocardial infarction. National Heart Attack Alert Program Coordinating Committee, 60 Minutes to Treatment Working Group. *Annals of Emergency Medicine* **23**: 311–29.

National Institute for Clinical Excellence (2002) *Guidance on the Use of Drugs for Early Thrombolysis in the Treatment of Acute Myocardial Infarction.* Technology appraisal No. 52. London: NICE.

Norris RM (1998) Fatality outside hospital from acute coronary events in three British health districts, 1994–5. United Kingdom Heart Attack Study Collaborative Group. *British Medical Journal* **316**: 1065–70.

O'Malley P, Favoloro R, Anderson B et al. (1991) Critical care nurse perceptions of family needs. *Heart and Lung* **20**: 189–201.

Papouchado M, Cox H, Bailey J et al. (2001) Early experience with transmission of data from moving ambulances to improve the care of patients with myocardial infarction. *Journal of Telemedicine and Telecare* **7**(suppl 1): 27–8.

Pedley D, Bissett K, Connolly E et al. (2003) Prospective observational cohort study of time saved by prehospital thrombolysis for ST elevation myocardial infarction delivered by paramedics. *British Medical Journal* **327**: 22–6.

Quinn T (1998) *Myocardial infarction in PDNT Book 1: Cardiology*. London: Emap Healthcare.

Quinn T, Morse T (2003) The interdisciplinary interface in managing patients with suspected cardiac pain. *Emergency Nurse* **11**: 22–4.

Quinn T, Thompson DR (1995) Administration of thrombolytic therapy to patients with acute myocardial infarction. *Accident and Emergency Nursing* **3**: 208–14.

Quinn T, Whitbread M (2005) Reduction of treatment delay in patients with ST-elevation myocardial infarction: impact of pre-hospital diagnosis and direct referral to primary percutaneous intervention. *European Heart Journal* **26**: 1343.

Quinn T, Butters A, Todd I (2002) Implementing paramedic thrombolysis: an overview. *Accident and Emergency Nursing* **10**: 189–96.

Quinn T, Dickson R, Jayram R et al. (2005a) *Describing the experience of patients and perceptions of members of the health care team in hospitals engaged in the British Heart Foundation acute coronary syndrome (ACS) nurse pilot project*. Final report to the Steering Group. London: British Heart Foundation.

Quinn T, Weston C, Birkhead J et al. (2005b) Redefining the coronary care unit: an observational study of patients admitted to hospital in England and Wales in 2003. *Quarterly Journal of Medicine* **98**: 797–802.

Quinn T, Minard D, Thayne R et al. (2006) Improving emergency cardiac care in a high performance ambulance service: the Staffordshire experience. *British Journal of Cardiology* in press.

Rawles J (1997) Quantification of the benefit of earlier thrombolytic therapy: five-year results of the Grampian Region Early Anistreplase Trial (GREAT). *Journal of the American College of Cardiology* **30**: 1181–6.

Rawles J, Kenmure ACF (1980) The coronary care controversy. *British Medical Journal* **281**: 783–6.

Sabatine M, Cannon C, Gibson C (2005) Addition of clopidogrel to aspirin and fibrinolytic therapy for acute myocardial infarction with ST segment elevation. *New England Journal of Medicine* **352**: 1179–89.

Savonitto S, Armstrong P, Lincoff A et al. (2003) Risk of intracranial haemorrhage with combined fibrinolytic and glycoprotein IIb/IIIa inhibitor therapy in acute myocardial infarction. *European Heart Journal* **24**: 1807–14.

Sayer J, Archbold R, Wilkinson P et al. (2000) Prognostic implications of ventricular fibrillation in acute myocardial infarction: new strategies required for further mortality reduction. *Heart* **84**: 258–61.

Schofield P (2005) Acute myocardial infarction: the case for pre-hospital thrombolysis with or without percutaneous coronary intervention. *Heart* **91**(suppl III) iii7–11.

Scottish Executive Health Department (2002) *Coronary Heart Disease and Stroke Strategy for Scotland*. Edinburgh: The Stationery Office.

Solomon SD, Ridker PM, Antman E (1993) Ventricular arrhythmias in trials of thrombolytic therapy for acute myocardial infarction. A meta-analysis. *Circulation* **88**: 2575–81.

Stephenson D, Wardrope J, Goodacre S (2002) Is prehospital thrombolysis for acute myocardial infarction warranted in the urban setting? The case against. *Emergency Medicine Journal* **19**: 444–8.

Stringer K (1998) TIMI grade flow, mortality and the GUSTO III trial. *Pharmacotherapy* **18**: 699–705.

Svensson L, Axelsson C, Norlander R et al. (2004) Prognostic value of biochemical markers, 12 lead ECG and patient characteristics amongst patients calling for an ambulance due to a suspected acute coronary syndrome. *Journal of Internal Medicine* **255**: 469–77.

Terkelsen C, Lassen J, Norgaard B et al. (2004) Are we underestimating the full potential of early thrombolytic treatment in patients with acute myocardial infarction? *Heart* **89**: 483–4.

Terkelsen C, Lassen J, Norgaard B et al. (2005) Mortality rates in patients with ST-elevation vs non-ST-elevation acute myocardial infarction: observations from an unselected cohort. *European Heart Journal* **26**: 18–26.

Townend J, Doshi S (2005) Reducing mortality in myocardial infarction. *British Medical Journal* **330**: 856–7.

Unal B, Critchley J, Capewell S (2004) Explaining the decline in coronary heart disease mortality in England and Wales between 1981 and 2000. *Circulation* **109**: 1101–17.

Van de Werf F, Ardissino D, Betriu A et al. (2003) Management of acute myocardial infarction in patients presenting with ST-segment elevation. The Task Force on the Management of Acute Myocardial Infarction of the European Society of Cardiology. *European Heart Journal* **24**: 28–66.

Whitbread M, Leah V, Bell T et al. (2002) Recognition of ST elevation by paramedics. *Emergency Medicine Journal* **19**: 66–7.

Woollard M, Quinn T (2005) *Acute Coronary Syndromes. Ambulance Paramedic Training Manua*l. London: Edexcel.

Woollard M, Pitt K, Hayward A, et al. (2005) Limited benefits of ambulance telemetry in delivering early thrombolysis: a randomised controlled trial. *Emergency Medicine Journal* **22**: 209–15.

8 Heart failure

MARK GRETTON

Heart failure is one of the more poorly understood cardiac conditions. Whereas laypeople generally have an idea of what a heart attack is and some understanding of the term 'cardiac arrest', they are often completely ignorant of heart failure in both causes and presentation. A recent study found that only 3% of almost 8000 randomly selected people from 9 European countries could identify heart failure from a description of typical symptoms (Spurgeon 2005). This is perhaps surprising, given both the prevalence of the condition and the very poor prognosis that it often carries. Survival rates are worse than those for breast and prostate cancer and there is a high risk of sudden death, often as a result of cardiac arrhythmias. Despite this, it is probable that, although members of the lay public would have a good understanding of breast cancer and some understanding of prostate cancer, they may be almost completely ignorant of heart failure. It is perhaps not unfair to say that this lack of understanding can also be found in health professionals.

It is estimated that there are around 65 000 new cases per year of heart failure. Officially recorded deaths suggest that there are around 11 000 deaths per annum from heart failure, but this is likely to be a gross underestimation. Death certificates explicitly guide doctors that heart failure is a mode of death rather than a cause of death and it is likely that this leads doctors to noting coronary heart disease rather than heart failure as the cause of death. Given that other data show that 40% of heart failure sufferers die within 1 year of the diagnosis, it is likely that a more accurate figure would be 24 000 deaths per year, equating to around 4% of all deaths in the UK in a year (British Heart Foundation 2005).

Studies that have attempted to assess the prevalence of heart failure in populations have not been uniform in their description of heart failure, some considering that it is proved if the ejection fraction – the percentage of blood ejected from the left ventricle on each contraction – is below 40%, some positing below 30% whereas others prefer to focus on clinical factors such as breathlessness, exercise intolerance and fluid retention. In the light of this, it is probable that the overall prevalence of heart failure is 3–20/1000 population, although this exceeds 100/1000 in those aged 65 years and over (Davis et

Cardiac Care: An Introduction for Healthcare Professionals. Edited by David Barrett, Mark Gretton and Tom Quinn
© 2006 John Wiley & Sons Ltd

al. 2000). Paradoxically, there may be increasing numbers of people with heart failure as more effective treatments for heart attacks mean that an increasing number of people are surviving to suffer ventricular dysfunction.

As heart failure carries a worse quality of life than most other common medical conditions, psychological problems are common, with over a third of people with the condition experiencing severe and prolonged depressive illness. This adds up to a considerable cost to the health service, because heart failure accounts for about 50% of all cardiac admissions and re-admission rates can be as high as 50% over 3 months. It has been estimated that half of these re-admissions may be preventable (Department of Health or DH 2000).

In this chapter I look at definitions of heart failure and the complex pathological processes that make up this condition. I also look at the presentation of heart failure, focusing on the difficulties that are sometimes present in diagnosis, and examine the treatment that the person with a failing heart will need.

DEFINITIONS OF HEART FAILURE

The exact prevalence and incidence of heart failure in a population can be difficult to determine because there is no classically agreed definition of heart failure. Attempts at definition have focused either on the underpinning pathophysiological changes such as the inability of the heart to pump blood at a rate adequate to supply the organs and tissues with oxygen or, more pragmatically, on the associated symptoms caused by ventricular dysfunction (Davis et al. 2000). Further confusion has been caused by the more recent 'discovery' of diastolic heart failure, when the heart fails despite no loss in systolic function. In spite of these difficulties, a helpful definition is 'the inability of the heart to pump sufficient blood forward to meet the metabolic demands of the body or the ability to do so only if the cardiac filling pressures are problematically high causing a "backing up" of pressure or both'. It is useful at this point to consider some subdivisions of heart failure and what is normally meant by these terms.

Forward failure

This is the inability of the heart to pump blood to the tissues and organs of the body, leading to a problematic decrease in organ perfusion, as a result of decreased cardiac output (Braunwald 1992).

Backward failure

This is the inability of the ventricle to pump its volume of blood, resulting in an accumulation of blood that causes a rise in the pressure in the ventricle, which then 'backs up' into the atrium and the venous system (Braunwald 1992).

Systolic failure

Classically, most heart failure has been considered to be systolic failure, which describes the impaired pump function that results in a reduced ejection fraction and an enlarged left ventricle with increased pooling of blood. This may have been caused by myocardial infarction (MI) or some unknown cause such as dilated cardiomyopathy.

Diastolic failure

This refers to what may be a sizable minority of patients who present with symptoms of heart failure but, on investigation, show no evidence of ventricular systolic dysfunction or acute valvular incompetence. Diagnosis is made by ruling out other causes of cardiac dysfunction and other conditions that may masquerade as heart failure (National Institute for Clinical Excellence or NICE 2003).

Acute heart failure

This describes heart failure occurring secondary to a sudden and traumatic insult to the heart such as an MI or acute valvular dysfunction, whereby the sympathetic compensatory mechanisms of the body are unable to cope with the fall in cardiac output, which may rapidly lead to pulmonary oedema and circulatory collapse.

Chronic heart failure

This can develop over time, as the body progressively fails to compensate for the failure of the heart to pump adequately. It may have been initially caused by an MI, but could also be caused by valve disease or chronic hypertension (Laurent-Bopp 2000).

Left ventricular failure (LVF)

The left and right sides of the heart are separate from each other and can fail independently, but in practice it is rare for left-sided heart failure not to lead to right-sided failure. When the left ventricle fails, cardiac output falls and organs and tissues become poorly perfused (forward failure), and the accumulation of blood in the left ventricle causes an increase in pressure in the left atrium and the pulmonary vascular circulation (backward failure), which may lead to pulmonary oedema (Laurent-Bopp 2000).

Right ventricular failure (RVF)

The right side of the heart may fail independently, though this is rare; more commonly the right ventricle fails because of LVF, as the backing up of pressure in the lungs starts to affect the right ventricle. The right ventricle may fail independently as a result of MI affecting predominantly the right ventricle, or of any lung condition causing increased pulmonary pressures that will eventually impair the functioning of the right ventricle. These include chronic obstructive pulmonary diseases such as asthma, emphysema and bronchitis, and pulmonary embolism. When the right ventricle fails, it is unable to discharge its blood volume to the lungs (forward failure) and the accumulation of blood backs up into the right atrium and the venous circulation, causing peripheral oedema (backward failure).

Cor pulmonale

This is a term used to denote right-sided heart failure that is secondary to a primary lung problem causing pulmonary hypertension (Weitzenblum 2003). This is a term that is perhaps less commonly used than it was 20 years ago.

Biventricular failure

This is when both ventricles fail during heart failure. It is common if LVF is untreated for the right ventricle then to fail.

Congestive cardiac failure

This is a term used to indicate heart failure involving both sides of the heart and characterised by breathlessness resulting from pulmonary oedema. Although this term is widely used by health professionals, some specialists believe that it is essentially meaningless in describing the clinical syndrome of heart failure.

PATHOPHYSIOLOGY

Causes of heart failure are many and various, but most sufferers in the UK whom the health professional will encounter will have myocardial dysfunction as the underlying disorder of heart failure. This is most likely to be caused by an MI, but can also be caused by primary heart muscle problems (i.e. cardiomyopathy), hypertension, valvular incompetence or stenosis, cardiac arrhythmias of any cause, toxins (such as alcohol), thyrotoxicosis or more rarely the tropical malady beri-beri (Laurent-Bopp 2000). As the heart fails as a result of one or more of these factors, the left ventricle loses its ability to pump effectively, causing tissues and organs to be starved of nutrients. The volume of blood in the left ventricle at the end of diastole increases and so the pressure in the left ventricle increases. In turn this causes an increase in pressure in the left atrium and the pulmonary venous system. Increased pulmonary capillary hydrostatic pressure can then lead to the movement of fluid from the pulmonary vasculature into the alveoli, producing pulmonary oedema (Mattu 2003).

Subsequent to this the right ventricle may fail, as it struggles against the increased pulmonary pressure. Pressure will increase in the right ventricle and then in the right atrium and back into the venous circulation. As hydrostatic pressure increases in the vascular system fluid may move into the interstitial space, causing peripheral oedema.

This understanding of heart failure held sway until the 1980s, because it seemed to explain the presenting symptoms of 'congestive heart failure' well: the fatigue of the patient caused by forward failure as the left ventricle struggled to propel sufficient oxygenated blood to the tissues and organs, the breathlessness as pressure increased in the left atrium and the pulmonary veins causing a movement of fluid into the alveoli, and the pressure building up in the right ventricle and right atrium until it impeded venous drainage to the right side of the heart, causing peripheral oedema. In the last 20 years, and most dramatically in the last 10 years, has come an understanding that, although this model is persuasive, it is incomplete, and that the specific changes wrought by neurohormonal factors have a decisive impact on the progress of heart failure in an individual.

NEUROHORMONAL CHANGES IN HEART FAILURE

The neurohormonal changes that have some effect on heart failure are various and complicated, but it is useful to outline the key changes. Collectively, neurohormonal factors trigger a number of compensatory mechanisms that aim to improve the mechanical functioning of the heart. Thus, as myocardial dysfunction develops it leads to a fall in cardiac output and a drop in blood pressure that triggers baro(pressure) receptors in the aorta and the carotid sinus. This activates the sympathetic nervous system, which attempts to maintain cardiac output with an increase in heart rate, increased myocardial contractility and peripheral vasoconstriction (increased catecholamines). Unfortunately, beyond a certain point this puts an increasing strain on an already damaged heart as myocardial workload and oxygen demand are increased in an attempt to power these changes.

Activation of the renin–angiotensin–aldosterone system also results in vasoconstriction (angiotensin) and an increase in blood volume, with retention of salt and water (aldosterone) (Jackson et al. 2000). The body is here responding to a perceived loss of circulating fluid by attempting to ensure that there is no fluid loss through the renal system, so the sodium and water retention expands the plasma volume and increases preload, the volume of blood in the ventricle just before systole. This puts further strain on the heart as it struggles to move the increased volume of blood returning to it.

If the heart is failing, as is often the case, as a result of MI, the neurohormonal changes described above often lead to ventricular remodelling. This is a process whereby the infarcted, damaged segment of the myocardium becomes thinner and dilates, whereas the uninfarcted area around it changes shape, becoming generally more spherical. Thus, there is an increased likelihood of blood pooling in a ventricle that is less able to shift it, leading to a further reduction in cardiac output accompanied by the risk of clot formation within the ventricle.

A further development in our understanding of heart failure is in the role of diastolic dysfunction. Diastolic dysfunction comes from an increase in ventricular stiffness, leading to a reduction in ventricular compliance and a consequent reduction in ventricular filling. Causes of this may be left ventricular damage caused by hypertension or coronary heart disease. Diastolic failure is not without controversy; some estimates suggest that between 30 and 40% of people with heart failure have normal systolic function (Vasan et al. 1995) whereas others have effectively cast doubt on whether it exists, given the difficulty of differentiating the diagnosis from other conditions causing breathlessness and related symptoms (Caruana et al. 2000). Nevertheless, for people with breathlessness for which other causes have been ruled out it should be considered a diagnostic possibility.

DIAGNOSIS OF HEART FAILURE

As discussed earlier, the symptoms of heart failure are perhaps not as widely known among the lay public as other common cardiac conditions such as heart attack or angina, which may mean that sufferers are less likely to recognise symptoms of heart failure for what they are. There is no 'silver bullet' diagnostic test for heart failure; its diagnosis depends on sound clinical judgement based on a combination of the signs and symptoms present in heart failure and some specific tests. Although diagnosis is the province of doctors, other health professionals who may see the patient first should be able to glean valuable information from carefully assessing the patient. The New York Heart Association classification (Table 8.1) provides a functional classification of heart failure that is easy to use when assessing patients.

The principal symptoms of heart failure are breathlessness, fatigue, exercise intolerance and fluid retention. If a hospital patient who had just had a heart attack suddenly presented with these symptoms, a diagnosis of acute heart failure might be made with little difficulty. But although these symptoms are almost always present in heart failure, they are by no means limited to heart

Table 8.1 New York Heart Association classification of heart failure

Class	Description
I (mild)	No limitation of physical activity. Ordinary physical activity does not cause undue fatigue, palpitation or breathlessness
II (mild)	Slight limitation of physical activity. Comfortable at rest, but ordinary physical activity results in fatigue, palpitation or breathlessness
III (moderate)	Marked limitation of physical activity. Comfortable at rest, but less than ordinary activity causes fatigue, palpitation or breathlessness
IV (severe)	Unable to carry out any physical activity without discomfort. Symptoms of cardiac insufficiency at rest. If any physical activity is undertaken, discomfort is increased

failure alone. The following gives some other conditions that may mimic heart failure:

- Obesity
- Lung conditions, e.g. bronchitis, asthma, emphysema, pulmonary embolism
- Rib injury
- Drug-induced ankle swelling, e.g. non-steroidal anti-inflammatory drugs (NSAIDs), some calcium channel blockers
- Kidney disease
- Anxiety and depression
- Anaemia
- Thyroid disorders.

Blood pressure may be elevated in the early stages of acute heart failure, but will later drop and tend to be low in chronic heart failure. A useful examination tool may be to check for a displaced apex beat; normally the beat of the heart can be heard most clearly over the area where the V5 or V6 electrode may be placed for recording ECGs, but in heart failure it may well be displaced laterally, as a result of the increase in size of the left ventricle. When the apex beat is auscultated, a third heart sound may be heard, indicating a problem with ventricular filling, or sometimes a fourth heart sound, which may denote altered ventricular compliance. Displaced apex beats and extra heart sounds are more useful when detected along with other signs; in isolation they may be less reliable. Raised jugular venous pressure is a good predictor of heart failure, but is often not present (NICE 2003).

A chest X-ray is an important diagnostic test in heart failure. It can show whether the heart is enlarged and if there is pulmonary oedema secondary to LVF. A normal chest X-ray does not exclude the possibility of heart failure. An ECG should be recorded as soon as possible. Although there is no specific ECG abnormality associated with heart failure, there may be a number of important indicators:

- Is there evidence of recent MI?
- If the patient is known to have had a recent MI, is there evidence of re-occlusion?
- Is there any unusual arrhythmia?
- Is the patient tachycardic?

These may all be pointers towards heart failure. Equally importantly, if the ECG is entirely normal, it is highly unlikely that the patient's symptoms are the result of heart failure and an alternative explanation can be sought (Houghton et al. 1997).

The most useful blood test for detecting heart failure is to look for elevated levels of brain (or B-type) natriuretic peptides (BNPs). These are hormones that are stored in cardiac tissue and secreted from the ventricles, where they play an important role in moderating the effects of heart failure by counter-acting neurohormonal effects of vasoconstriction and sodium retention, and promoting diuresis and natriuresis. They have been shown to be sensitive to reduced left ventricular ejection fraction (LVEF), increased left ventricular volume and MI, and to be present in the blood in larger quantities in these conditions. As such they may be useful predictors of heart failure, although they may be significantly lower in obese people and significantly higher in women and all people aged over 60 (Hunt et al. 2005). As with the ECG, BNP levels are very sensitive negative predictors of heart failure; if the levels are normal it is highly unlikely that the patient is in heart failure (NICE 2003).

The most valuable test may be echocardiography, which can be regarded as the gold standard test for heart failure. This two-dimensional Doppler study of the heart can measure the ejection fraction, show whether portions of the ventricles are akinetic, demonstrate valvular incompetency and regurgitation, and detect whether any clots have formed in the ventricles. If a patient with symptoms of heart failure has an abnormal ECG or abnormal BNP result, echocardiography should be performed (NICE 2003).

TREATMENT OF HEART FAILURE

The aims of the treatment of heart failure are to improve first life expectancy and then quality of life (NICE 2003). Health practitioners' experience of heart failure will vary considerably depending on whether they are dealing with an acute episode in a hospital environment or a chronic episode in a community setting. Although there will inevitably be some treatment overlap, it is helpful to consider the two situations separately.

ACUTE HEART FAILURE IN THE HOSPITAL SETTING

The patient needs to be immediately linked to a cardiac monitor. Arrhythmias may reduce cardiac output and may need to be treated aggressively; in addition some prescribed therapeutic drugs may increase the risk of arrhythmias. Breathlessness should be treated with high-concentration oxygen, assuming that there is no history of chronic chest problems. If the patient's breathing is severely compromised mechanical ventilation may be needed. Non-invasive ventilation may also be tried. Diamorphine or morphine should be given to help calm the patient, steady the breathing and reduce the blood flow back to the heart, so reducing oxygen demand resulting from preload. The blood pressure should be monitored frequently and a urinary catheter may be inserted to monitor urinary output.

Invasive monitoring, such as central venous pressure (CVP) monitoring or pulmonary artery wedge pressure (PAWP) monitoring that give continuous indirect pressure monitoring within the heart chambers, may be instituted. This allows treatment to be titrated against pressure changes within the heart. An infusion of intravenous nitrate may be started. Nitrates are potent coronary vasodilators and also dilate the peripheral circulation, so they reduce the strain on the heart by reducing afterload (the force that the heart has to exert to move blood round the body) and preload. Caution needs to be exercised with nitrate administration in order to ensure that the patient does not become dangerously hypotensive. If the patient is shown to be fluid overloaded or to be in pulmonary oedema, the intake of fluids might have to be restricted and a diuretic such as furosemide may be given intravenously. Furosemide has a vasodilatory as well as a diuretic effect and, although useful, extreme caution must be taken to ensure that the patient does not become dehydrated. If it is believed that there is a significant element of right-sided heart failure, diuretics may be harmful because they may reduce normal left ventricular pressures problematically. Caution and effective monitoring are of paramount importance.

If the patient is hypotensive, inotropic drugs such as dobutamine and dopamine may be considered. These drugs increase myocardial contractility so they may increase the ejection fraction and improve cardiac output. Caution must be exercised because these drugs also cause peripheral vasoconstriction, which may increase afterload and increase the strain on the heart; this, coupled with the increased contractility as the heart is 'flogged' by the drug, may prove harmful as oxygen demand is increased (Laurent-Bopp and Shinn 2000). For this reason more powerful inotropic drugs such as adrenaline (epinephrine) and noradrenaline (norepinephrine) are avoided in acute heart failure by many clinicians because the inotropic benefits are outweighed by the increased myocardial strain.

If the patient does not respond to medical measures, interventions such as angioplasty or coronary artery bypass grafting (CABG) may be considered. If such an intervention is possible, the patient may be supported before and after the intervention with an intra-aortic balloon pump, whereby a catheter is inserted into the femoral artery and fed round to the arch of the aorta, where a helium balloon is repeatedly inflated and deflated. This improves cardiac output in systole and coronary artery filling in diastole.

Throughout an acute episode of heart failure, a patient is likely to be extremely anxious, frightened and uncomfortable. If the patient is hypoxic this may compound the agitation. It is imperative that the health professional be calm, sympathetic and reassuring, and explain carefully all the interventions and their rationale as clearly as possible. If patients are thirsty, they may benefit from sucking ice rather than drinking copiously. Patients may feel alternately too hot and too cold and carers must be alert to these changes and imaginative in dealing with them. Patients may find it very difficult to be comfortable, but may find breathing easier if sat upright. Even if their blood pressure is low and their pressure areas are at risk, it is generally best to assist patients to a position that is comfortable to them while encouraging regular movement and monitoring them closely.

CHRONIC HEART FAILURE

The treatment for the patient in chronic heart failure is predominantly drug based, but it is imperative that other factors are not neglected. Given that heart failure patients are often short of breath, tired and uncomfortable, it is not uncommon that they become depressed. Anxiety over progress and prognosis is common, and sometimes patients have problematic side effects from the drug regimen. It is important that the health professional helps patients to engage with their treatment, so that they understand why they are receiving it and what benefits it should bring them. This is particularly important if patients have been given dietary advice that may require them to alter their current eating and drinking habits. Patients should also be encouraged to voice any concerns about their progress and drug side effects, because they need to know that there are alternatives to the treatment that they are currently receiving. The NICE has sponsored a guideline to best practice in the management of chronic heart failure and this guideline underpins this section (NICE 2003).

Drug therapy

Diuretics have been the traditional mainstay of chronic heart failure for decades and their role in symptomatic relief remains important, current advice being that they should be used routinely to relieve symptoms of breathlessness and fluid retention, and titrated according to symptoms once other therapies such as ACE (angiotensin-converting enzyme) inhibitors and β blockers have been initiated (NICE 2003). The most commonly used diuretics are furosemide and bumetanide, which are loop diuretics, powerful drugs that affect the loop of Henle in the kidneys. Thiazide diuretics, such as bendroflumethiazide, act predominantly on the beginning of the distal tubule in the kidneys and may also be used. Spironolactone, which is a synthetic steroid, has an aldosterone-blocking action and as such also has a diuretic effect

(Hopkins 1999). This may be added in to other therapies if the patient still has symptoms of breathlessness and fluid retention. Some diuretics cause a lowering of the serum potassium, so the patient's biochemical profile should be regularly checked. The risk of low potassium is reduced if the patient is also taking an ACE inhibitor.

All patients with heart failure believed to be caused by systolic dysfunction should be considered for ACE inhibitors (NICE 2003). Clinical trials have demonstrated that they increase life expectancy and reduce hospital admission for this patient group (Flather et al. 2000). ACE inhibitors work by blocking the conversion of angiotensin I to angiotensin II. As described earlier, angiotensin II causes vasoconstriction in an attempt to maintain blood pressure in a failing heart, but this can put undue strain on the damaged myocardium and lead, after a heart attack, to ventricular remodelling. ACE inhibitors effectively have a vasodilatory effect that can prevent myocardial strain and remodelling. They include drugs such as captopril, enalapril and ramipril. These drugs should be started at a low dose to ensure patient tolerance and then increased to the maximum therapeutic level.

The vasodilatory effect can cause an initial drop in blood pressure, which can be accompanied by dizziness and patients should ideally be monitored while they have the initial dose. If this persists, an alternative ACE inhibitor may be tried. A frequent unwanted side effect of ACE inhibitors is a dry cough (sometimes referred to as 'captopril cough'). Generally speaking this is not sufficiently problematic to stop the prescription, and initially patients should be encouraged to persevere. If the cough becomes really troublesome, patients may be prescribed an angiotensin II receptor blocker as an alternative, such as valsartan or losartan (NICE 2003). These are a newer class of drug that have much the same effect as ACE inhibitors but with fewer side effects, including coughing (Kirk 1999). As a general rule ACE inhibitors are well tolerated and extremely beneficial to the patient in heart failure. Stopping ACE inhibitors in such patients is often associated with an increase in symptoms, so patients should be encouraged to persevere with this therapy and urged not to discontinue it except on specialist advice (NICE 2003).

Large clinical trials have shown that β blockers improve life expectancy in patients with heart failure caused by systolic dysfunction and reduce hospital admissions for these patients (Bouzamondo et al. 2001, Brophy et al. 2001). β Blockers have traditionally been avoided in heart failure, because it was felt that their undoubted negative inotropic effect would reduce cardiac output to a problematic degree. It is now known that the problematic neurohormonal activity in heart failure can be reduced by β blockers. Noradrenaline has been particularly implicated in heart failure as a cause of both increasing left ventricular dysfunction and the malignant tachyarrhythmias that lead to sudden cardiac death (SCD), and some β blockers have been shown to ameliorate these effects.

Not all β blockers may be effective, and research into this area continues. Nevertheless, it is clear that β blockers such as carvedilol and metoprolol are useful and the current advice is that such β blockers should be added carefully to therapy ('start low and go slow') after ACE inhibitors and diuretics, even if symptoms are controlled with those drugs (NICE 2003). Health professionals need to be aware that β blockers do have side effects, and patients need to be aware of them and to report them. This is particularly important if the patient notices becoming more tired, weak or breathless and showing a persistent weight gain. These symptoms may be the result of the patient getting accustomed to the drug, but they may be caused by the drug exacerbating the patient's condition, so the patient must be encouraged to report such symptoms to a specialist as soon as possible. Patients should be encouraged to weigh themselves regularly at the same time each day. It is important too that patients realise that β blockers are prescribed principally for their effect on survival rather than for the relief of symptoms, and that any symptomatic relief that they do get may be gradual over a period of months (NICE 2003). Patients often report other unpleasant effects of β blockers, such as nausea, headaches, diarrhoea and cold extremities (see www.drugtalk.com) and it is important that they are aware that the drugs are helping them, sometimes despite appearances. Again, patients should be urged to persevere with β blockers and not to stop taking them unless they have agreed this with a specialist.

Other drugs used to manage heart failure will largely depend on whether the sufferer has any other problems, such as arrhythmias or a high serum cholesterol, that need to be managed together with the heart failure. Digoxin may be added in to the therapies, if diuretics, ACE inhibitors and β blockers are not controlling the condition, or may be added earlier if the patient has atrial fibrillation, which may reduce cardiac output caused by the loss of contraction from the atria. Aspirin is recommended for patients in heart failure with coronary heart disease, although doubt has been cast in some quarters as to whether it may limit the beneficial effects of ACE inhibitors (Cleland 2002). Further information about the cardiac medication used to treat heart failure can be found in Chapter 13.

LIFESTYLE FACTORS

There is little hard evidence from randomised controlled studies to guide patients on modification of lifestyle factors (NICE 2003). Nevertheless, there are some areas on which there is consensus about what is considered to be best practice and the health professional caring for a person with heart failure will be expected to provide advice in these areas. If patients smoke they should be strongly encouraged to stop, and supported as far as is possible.

Drinking alcohol has been shown to damage heart muscle if carried out to excess (Piano 2002) and anyone with heart failure secondary to alcoholic heart disease should be strongly urged to stop drinking (NICE 2003). In heart failure from other causes, such as after an MI, patients may need to be warned about the potential risks of taking in large amounts of fluids if they drink beer, lager or cider. Despite this, there is plenty of anecdotal evidence of people with heart failure continuing to drink alcohol without ill-effects, and this should be borne in mind when advising patients. There is no evidence that people with heart failure should be routinely advised to stop drinking, and of course it must be remembered that there is evidence that people who have stopped drinking after suffering a heart attack have been at increased risk of further fatal and non-fatal heart attacks compared with those who have continued drinking (Jackson et al. 1991) and that the general protective effect of alcohol for MI is well established (Jackson et al. 1991, Woodward and Tunstall-Pedoe 1995, McElduff and Dobson 1997).

Patients are often encouraged to restrict their fluid intakes and to reduce their sodium levels by removing salt from their diet, in the belief that this will reduce fluid retention and breathlessness. There is no compelling evidence that this is the case, and any benefits need to be set against the risk of dehydrating the patient and causing a lack of appetite by making food unpalatable. If the patient is obese, a weight reduction diet may be appropriate because this may help reduce breathlessness.

Patients should be encouraged to exercise if they so wish and to discover their own limits. Both aerobic exercise, such as brisk walking, cycling and swimming, and resistive exercise, such as weight-training, have been shown to reduce symptoms and improve the quality of life without damaging cardiac function, although there are currently no proven long-term benefits (Rees et al. 2004).

Patients with heart failure can normally drive, although if they are HGV (heavy goods vehicle) or PSV (passenger service vehicle) licence holders they should be advised to contact the Driver and Vehicle Licensing Agency for advice, because they may be prohibited from driving an HGV or PSV. If this proves to be the case, patients will need support and advice regarding their job occupations. There is no reason for someone with heart failure not to use a commercial passenger aircraft if he or she so wishes.

Sexual activity may be compromised by heart failure, as a result of symptoms of fatigue and breathlessness and concern from both the patient and partner about whether any further harm will be caused. In addition, erectile dysfunction has been reported in some medications used in heart failure such as β blockers and diuretics. The health professional should be prepared to talk to the patient about these issues and be willing to initiate conversations, because it is unlikely that patients will raise such issues themselves.

Anxiety and depression are common among people with heart failure and the health professional should be alert for signs of this and be prepared to talk to the patient and suggest ways of dealing with them. It may be that they are related to symptoms or anxiety over job or sexual performance, and possible solutions can be suggested. Some patients may benefit from professional counselling or antidepressant drugs. Patients do need to be advised that, if they take St John's wort for depression, this may reduce the efficacy of some prescribed drugs, such as digoxin and warfarin (NICE 2003).

If patients' symptoms are uncontrolled by their treatment and they become increasingly ill, it may be appropriate to refer them to the specialist symptom control team. In the past, nurses working out of such teams have tended to focus on patients with cancer, but increasingly they are widening their remit to support people with end-stage heart failure.

CONCLUSION

Heart failure is a problematic condition, in terms of both mortality and health-care cost. It is a complex syndrome of symptoms with a number of potential causes, although it is most often seen after a heart attack. Diagnosis may be difficult and needs careful and thorough examination. Classic early therapy to support the acutely failing heart consists of diuretics, nitrates and inotropes; in the chronic phase of heart failure, ACE inhibitors and β blockers are now first-line treatment. Heart failure is often frightening and depressing for the sufferer and the health professional must be aware of the emotional and psychological support that these people will need.

REFERENCES

Bouzamondo A, Hulot JS, Sanchez P et al. (2001) Beta-blocker treatment in heart failure. *Fundamental and Clinical Pharmacology* **15**: 95–109.

Braunwald E (1992) *A Textbook of Cardiovascular Medicine*. Philadelphia: WB Saunders.

British Heart Foundation (2005) *Mortality from Heart Failure*. Available from www.heartstats.org/datapage.asp?id=752

Brophy JM, Joseph L, Rouleau JL (2001) Beta-blockers in congestive heart failure. A Bayesian meta-analysis. *Annals of Internal Medicine* **134**: 550–560.

Caruana L, Petrie MC, Davie MP, McMurray JJV (2000) Do patients with suspected heart failure and preserved left ventricular systolic function suffer from 'diastolic heart failure' or from misdiagnosis? A prospective descriptive study. *British Medical Journal* **321**: 215–18.

Cleland JG (2002) Is aspirin 'the weakest link' in cardiovascular prophylaxis? The surprising lack of evidence supporting the use of aspirin for cardiovascular disease. *Progress in Cardiovascular Diseases* **44**: 275–92.

Davis RC, Hobbs FDR, Lip GYH (2000) ABC of heart failure: History and epidemiology. *British Medical Journal* **320**: 39–42.

Department of Health (2000) *National Service Framework for Coronary Heart Disease.* London: Department of Health.

Flather MD, Yusuf S, Kober L et al. (2000) Long term ACE inhibitor therapy in patients with heart failure or left ventricular dysfunction: a systematic overview of data from individual patients. ACE inhibitor myocardial infarction collaborative group. *Lancet* **355**: 1575–81.

Hopkins SJ (1999) *Drugs and Pharmacology for Nurses*, London: Churchill Livingstone.

Houghton AR, Sparrow NJ, Toms E, Cowley AJ (1997) Should general practitioners use the electrocardiogram to select patients for echocardiography? *International Journal of Cardiology* **62**: 31–6.

Hunt SA, Abraham WJ, Chin MH et al. (2005) *ACC/AHA guideline update for the diagnosis and management of chronic heart failure in the adult*. Available from www.acc.org/clinical/guidelines/failure/index.pdf

Jackson R, Scragg R, Beaglehole R (1991) Alcohol consumption and risk of coronary heart disease. *British Medical Journal* **303**: 211–16.

Jackson G, Gibbs CR, Davies MK, Lip GYH (2000) ABC of heart failure: Pathophysiology. *British Medical Journal* **320**: 167–70.

Kirk JK (1999) Angiotensin-II receptor antagonists: their place in therapy. *American Family Physician*. **59**: 11. Available from www.aafp.org/afp/990600ap/3140.html

Laurent-Bopp D (2000) Heart failure. In: Woods SL, Froelicher ESS, Motzer SU (eds), *Cardiac Nursing*, 4th edn. Philadelphia: Lippincott, pp 560–79.

Laurent-Bopp D, Shinn JA (2000) Shock. In: Woods SL, Froelicher ESS, Motzer SU (eds), *Cardiac Nursing*, 4th edn. Philadelphia: Lippincott, pp 614–38.

McElduff P, Dobson AJ (1997) How much alcohol and how often? Population based case-control study of alcohol consumption and risk of a major coronary event. *British Medical Journal* **314**: 1159–64.

Mattu A (2003) *Pulmonary Edema, Cardiogenic*. Available from www.emedicine.com/med/topic1955.htm

National Institute of Clinical Excellence (2003) *Chronic Heart Failure – National clinical guideline for diagnosis and management in primary and secondary care*. London: NICE.

Piano MR (2002) Alcoholic cardiomyopathy: incidence, clinical characteristics and pathophysiology. *Chest* **121**: 1638–50.

Rees K, Taylor RS, Singh S et al. (2004) Exercise based rehabilitation for heart failure. *The Cochrane Database of Systematic Reviews 2004*. Issue 3.

Remmes J, Miettinen H, Reunanen A, Pyorala K (1991) Validity of clinical diagnosis of heart failure in primary health care. *European Heart Journal*. **12**: 315–21.

Spurgeon D (2005) European public are unaware of heart failure symptoms. *British Medical Journal* **331**: 535.

Vasan RS, Benjamin EJ, Levy D (1995) Prevalence, clinical features and prognosis of diastolic heart failure: an epidemiologic perspective. *Journal of the American College of Cardiology* **26**: 1565–74.

Weitzenblum E (2003) Chronic cor pulmonale. *Heart* **89**: 225–30.

Woodward M, Tunstall-Pedoe H (1995) Alcohol consumption, diet, coronary risk factors, and prevalent coronary heart disease in men and women in the Scottish heart health study. *Journal of Epidemiology of Community Health* **49**: 354–62.

9 Arrhythmias

MARK GRETTON

An arrhythmia, sometimes referred to as a dysrhythmia, is an abnormality of the heart's rhythm. This may be the result of the heart beating unusually quickly, unusually slowly or in an irregular way. Someone with an arrhythmia may be completely unaware of it, or may experience palpitations or more serious symptoms such as breathlessness, chest pain, unconsciousness and even sudden cardiac death (SCD). Cardiac arrhythmia is believed to affect more than 700 000 people in England and is one of the 10 most common causes of a person needing hospital treatment (Department of Health or DH 2005). These admissions may be caused by arrhythmias secondary to an existing heart condition such as coronary heart disease (CHD), heart failure or cardiomyopathy, or they may result from inherited factors such as congenital heart disease.

The importance of cardiac arrhythmias has become increasingly recognised in recent years, as more cardiologists have specialised in arrhythmia management. This importance has been recognised by the government commissioning and recently publishing a chapter on arrhythmias to add to the National Service Framework for CHD (DH 2005). In this chapter I look at the pathophysiology of arrhythmias, the assessment of arrhythmias by cardiac monitoring, and the care, treatment and management of the person suffering a cardiac arrhythmia.

PATHOPHYSIOLOGY OF ARRHYTHMIAS

A normal sinus rhythm is considered to have a heart rate of between 60 and 99 beats/minute (bpm). A rate below 60 bpm is termed a 'bradycardia', a rate of 100 bpm or above a 'tachycardia'. It can be useful to classify bradycardias as absolute, when the heart rate is slower than 40 bpm, or relative, when the heart rate is unremarkable, but is inappropriately slow for the patient (Resuscitation Council (UK) 2005). Although these are predominantly descriptive terms and should not be understood as necessarily denoting a problematic abnormality, it is useful to consider cardiac arrhythmias as either brad-

Cardiac Care: An Introduction for Healthcare Professionals. Edited by David Barrett, Mark Gretton and Tom Quinn
© 2006 John Wiley & Sons Ltd

yarrhythmias or tachyarrhythmias. In the normally functioning heart, the cells that display the fastest intrinsic depolarisation rate are those of the sinoatrial (SA) node. These cells have a beat that pre-empts all other cells and suppresses their automaticity – their ability to fire off impulses spontaneously.

Although the SA node in the adult characteristically has a depolarisation rate of 60–99/minute, other areas of automaticity have slower rates. The atrioventricular (AV) node and the bundle of His have a rate of around 40–50 depolarisations/minute and the Purkinje system, which runs through the ventricles, has a rate of around 30–40/minute (Klabunde 2005a). Normally, these other areas of potential automaticity are suppressed by the SA node – a phenomenon known as overdrive suppression. Thus, the SA node is normally the dominant pacemaker in the heart, whereas other areas are latent pacemakers (Jacobson 2000). A deviation from this is called altered impulse formation and can cause either slow or fast heart rhythms

BRADYARRHYTHMIAS

Altered impulse formation occurs when a localised group of cells develops an intrinsic firing rate exceeding that of the SA node. This might happen if the rate of the SA node becomes suppressed, firing less frequently than normal. As a result a latent pacemaker may then become dominant and will fire, producing an escape beat or rhythm. Alternatively, the SA node rate may not slow, but one of the latent pacemakers may develop an intrinsic rate of depolarisation that is faster than the SA node, so this then becomes the dominant pacemaker, firing off impulses that produce an ectopic beat or rhythm (Smith and Kampine 1990). There are two mechanisms for altered impulse formation.

A neurohormonal mechanism refers to a change in the dynamics between the sympathetic (SNS) and parasympathetic nervous systems (PNS). The SNS of adrenaline (epinephrine) and noradrenaline (norepinephrine) increases automaticity. The PNS of cholinergic stimulation via the vagus nerve reduces the probability of pacemaker cells being open, so the firing rate is slowed. The SA node and the AV node are most sensitive to vagal stimulation, followed by atrial tissue, with ventricular tissue being the least sensitive. Moderate vagal stimulation can slow the sinus rate and move the pacemaker to another site. Strong vagal stimulation can completely suppress the SA and AV nodes and atrial tissue, resulting in the emergence of a ventricular escape rhythm as an alternative to the heart producing no impulses at all and becoming asystolic (Smith and Kampine 1990). Tissue injury can decrease the rate of impulse formation, as can ageing; it is not entirely clear why, although it is likely that ischaemia plays a part in this.

It is probable that the most common cause of bradyarrhythmias is conduction blocks. These are not alterations in the firing rate, but rather a blockade of impulses across the normal conduction pathways so that one part of the conduction pathway loses contact with the next (Da Costa et al. 2002). This may be caused by fibrosis, ischaemia or trauma. As a result of the blockage, the pacemaker function has to start from sites distal from the blockage. This may produce escape rhythms and heart block rhythms.

TACHYARRHYTHMIAS

There are three mechanisms causing tachyarrhythmias: increased automaticity, re-entrant rhythms and triggered activity (Smith and Kampine 1990). Increased automaticity is when cells fire off more rapidly than normal. These are generally pacemaker cells and so produce sinus, atrial or junctional tachycardias, depending on the area initiating the increased rate. Re-entrant rhythms occur when an impulse travels through an area of the myocardium, depolarises it and then re-enters the same area to depolarise it again (Jacobson 2000). For this to occur there has to be a unidirectional block, so that the impulse can conduct in one direction but not the other – in effect a short circuiting of the affected area is set up. In addition, there needs to be a slowing of the impulse as it travels back through the affected area, or the impulse will not be able to depolarise again but instead will just die out on the end of the previous impulse. This general concept is sometimes called micro-re-entry if it involves merely a small amount of tissue in the conduction system and macro-re-entry if the loop involves large tracts of tissue, such as occurs in AV bypass tracts (Julian et al. 2005). Re-entrant rhythms are thought to be the major cause of tachyarrhythmias and the mechanism for many lethal arrhythmias (Jacobson 2000).

Triggered activity refers to the state whereby cellular depolarisation can trigger a second action potential – in effect, where a cell may depolarise far earlier than it should. These are sometimes referred to as after-depolarisations and can be early or late. Early after-depolarisations occur during the depolarisation of the previous beat – what is termed the 'refractory period'. As the refractory period should, by definition, be a time when the cell is not depolarising, this can destabilise the cell and cause a series of rapid depolarisations. Late after-depolarisations occur when a cellular depolarisation has been complete, but before the next depolarisation would normally occur (Smith and Kampine 1990), again potentially disturbing the rhythm of the heart.

CARDIAC MONITORING – A SYSTEMATIC APPROACH

Before we look at specific arrhythmic states we need to be clear what we are looking for on the electrocardiogram (ECG) as it presents on a heart monitor, because cardiac monitoring may be the best way to detect what rhythm the heart is in. Most of us recognise heart rhythms in the way that we recognise everything else, by pattern recognition. We often do not need to analyse this too much, for example, I would not say 'Hmm, there's a woman walking into my house, she is attractive, dark-haired, staggering under the weight of a number of shopping bags, looking at me in irritation as I continue to sit reading the paper, so, on balance, this must be my wife' when I see my wife. We recognise people if we are familiar with what they look like. Similarly with ECG rhythms, the more we see them, the easier it is for us to recognise them at first glance. But it is useful to have a more systematic approach in mind for those that we do not recognise. The following method, suggested by the Resuscitation Council (UK), may be useful for rhythms with which we are not immediately familiar, strangers wandering into our lives.

SIX-STAGE APPROACH TO RHYTHM RECOGNITION (RESUSCITATION COUNCIL UK 2000)

1. Is there electrical activity?

When we talk of electrical activity and the ECG, we are referring to deviations from the baseline, either upwards or downwards. When there is no electrical activity, we really have only two situations: either an electrode has come loose or the patient is asystolic, with no electrical activity from the heart at all. You do not need to be an expert to see that it is important to understand quickly which situation you have and that the former is easier to put right than the latter.

This brings us to the most important law of ECG interpretation:

Treat the patient not the monitor.

If patients are reading the newspaper and talking to you, they are not asystolic. If they are slumped and motionless, immediately perform the ABCDE assessment. Another thing to remember is that a so-called 'straight line' or 'flat-line' asystole is generally no such thing, because closer examination will show that the line undulates, swinging slightly upwards then downwards. Truly straight lines are almost always artificially produced; nature likes to do curves. 'Flat liners' hardly ever are, no matter how exciting the film or how moodily Kiefer Sutherland stares into the camera.

2. Is the rate fast or slow?

The easiest way to discover the heart rate is to see what rate the monitor says it is. The safest is to check the patient's pulse and see if that matches what is shown on the machine. Another way is to print out a rhythm strip from the monitor and count out 30 large squares, then count the number of individual QRS complexes that are in those 30 squares. If you then multiply that number by 10 that will give you a good approximation of the heart rate. So, if there are 7 QRS complexes in the 30 squares, the heart rate will be around 70 bpm. Another way is to count the number of large squares between any two consecutive R waves (what is sometimes called the R–R interval). Then divide this figure into 300. So, if there are four large squares between two R waves, the rate is 75 bpm. This is probably the quickest DIY method and has the advantage that, once you become familiar with it, you do not have to do the calculation, you remember that 7 squares is 42, 6 is 50, 5 is 60, 4 is 75, 3 is 100, 2 is 150 and 1 is you anxiously commencing the ABCDE assessment as a rate of 300 bpm is normally not compatible with an effective cardiac output. You can be more accurate by selecting the R–R interval and dividing the number of small squares therein into 1500, but this is best left to numerical wizards or people with calculators.

3. Is the rhythm regular or irregular?

You can normally tell this just by looking, although the faster the heart rate the more difficult it can get. If in doubt, try turning up the sound volume on the monitor: our ears are often better than our eyes in differentiating between regular and irregular. If still in doubt, print off another rhythm strip and put a piece of paper against the rhythm strip so that you can put a mark on your paper opposite three of the R waves. Then move your piece of paper along the rhythm strip. If the marks still correspond with R waves, the rhythm is regular; if they do not, then it is not.

Irregular heart rhythms are sometimes caused by ventricular ectopics, broad, bizarre complexes on the ECG caused by an impulse arising outside the normal conduction pathway. These can be uncomfortable, but benign, particularly if all the ectopics are the same shape. These are sometimes called unifocal or monomorphic ventricular ectopics. If they have a number of different shapes, they may be multifocal or polymorphic, and these can be more problematic. You should always look for a cause for multifocal ventricular ectopics, such as chest pain or the patient suffering from a lack of oxygen. The other common reason for an irregular heart rhythm is if the patient has the rhythm of atrial fibrillation (AF), where the top chambers of the heart vibrate rapidly but only conduct a certain amount of impulses through to the ventricles. AF rarely causes a collapse and can sometimes be very well tolerated, but if it is new it always needs treating, because it carries a significant risk of stroke as a result of blood pooling and clotting in the non-contracting atria.

Patients with irregular heart rhythms may be symptom free. They may, on the other hand, be complaining of palpitations in the chest, chest pain or breathlessness. If they are, and particularly if they are having these symptoms for the first time, then they need to be reviewed by a specialist health professional.

4. Are the QRS complexes broad or narrow?

In normal conduction, the QRS complexes are narrow, i.e. they are generally only two to two and a half small squares across. In terms of time, this equates to 0.08–0.10 seconds. If they get to three small squares across or longer (≥0.12 seconds) when measured from their widest point, they are classified as broad and this is abnormal. It is generally caused by either a delay in conduction across the ventricles, such as a bundle-branch block, or most commonly by a rhythm starting in the ventricles, such as a ventricular tachycardia (VT). Either way it is unusual and should be reported, even if the patient is asymptomatic.

5. Are there P waves present?

P waves represent the movement of electricity across the atria that should precede the contraction of the atria. As such, you expect to see P waves in front of each QRS complex. If you do not, this is abnormal. If you can see no P waves at all, or each P wave is inverted (upside down), this may be the result of the impulse starting at the AV node instead of the SA node. If there are P waves some, but not all, of the time, this may be one of the types of heart block. Patients may be symptomatic in either of these situations, but even if they are not, these are significant findings that need reporting.

There may be no P waves if the patient has a broad complex tachycardia, because this is almost certainly a VT, a potentially lethal arrhythmia. Bear in mind that the faster a rhythm is the more difficult it is to detect P waves. As a useful rule of thumb, P waves are like most other things in life: if you do not think you can see them, then they probably are not there (Sally Waters 1987, personal communication).

6. Are the P waves correctly associated with the QRS complexes?

If there are P waves, then, as well as there being one for each QRS complex, we should expect the distance from the start of the P wave to the start of the QRS complex to be between three and five small squares (0.12–0.2 seconds). If the distance is any greater than this, there is some type of heart block present. Remember that you are measuring from the *start* of the P wave, not its *end*, as sometimes seems most logical to do. The nurse who first taught me about heart blocks confessed that for a while she had measured from the completion of the P wave to the QRS. As she told me: 'When I thought they were in block, they really WERE in block!'

If the distance is less than three small squares, this is a rarer but still important finding, because it may be indicative of a pre-excitation syndrome, where an accessory pathway bypasses part of the normal conduction system of the heart and speeds up conduction between the atria and ventricles. This can lead to tachycardias that are dangerous and sometimes lethal.

WHAT ARE WE LOOKING AT, THEN? PULLING IT ALL TOGETHER

What we get from all of the above depends on what we have found, rather obviously. But the value of this method is that, although we may not be able to put a name to a rhythm, we can, if we follow the six-stage approach, generally work out something useful from it. This helps us to decide whether we are dealing with something immediately problematic or have time to ponder. This is particularly useful if we are reporting a problem via the telephone to a senior colleague. We might say that we are not sure, but we think that it might be atrial fibrillation. And we might or might not be right. But if, instead, we say that the rate is between 140 and 170 bpm, the rhythm is irregular, the QRS complexes are narrow and there are no clear P waves to be seen, then, if the person on the other end of the phone does not recognise that as atrial fibrillation with a rapid ventricular response, we can conclude that the person knows less about cardiac monitoring than we do.

Of course, most of the time when you work through the six-stage approach to examine a heart rhythm, you will find that there is electrical activity, the rate is between 60 and 99 bpm, it is regular, the QRS complexes are narrow, there is a P wave associated with each QRS complex, and the start of the P waves is between three and five small squares from the QRS complexes. If this is the case, we are looking at a person who is in a normal sinus rhythm. Good for him or her!

EXAMPLES OF BRADYARRHYTHMIAS

SINUS BRADYCARDIA

Figure 9.1 shows a sinus bradycardia, because the QRS complexes are narrow and there is a P wave preceding each one. The distance from the start of the P wave to the start of the QRS is about four small squares (0.16 seconds), which is in the normal range and so rules out the possibility of this being heart block. The rate is interesting, being around 25 bpm. This is unusually slow for a healthy heart, but can be present in athletes with highly developed and efficient cardiovascular systems (Jensen-Urstad et al. 1997). Heart rates are generally slower in elderly people, so the age and fitness of the person would give us more idea of the cause of this arrhythmia. Other causes of sinus bradycardia include hypothermia and hypothyroidism, or overdosage of drugs such as verapamil or β blockers. Sinus bradycardia can also be a side effect of hypoxia.

FIRST-DEGREE HEART BLOCK

In Figure 9.2 we can see that the rate is about 75 bpm, so this is not a bradycardia. Given that the rhythm is regular and the QRS complexes are narrow

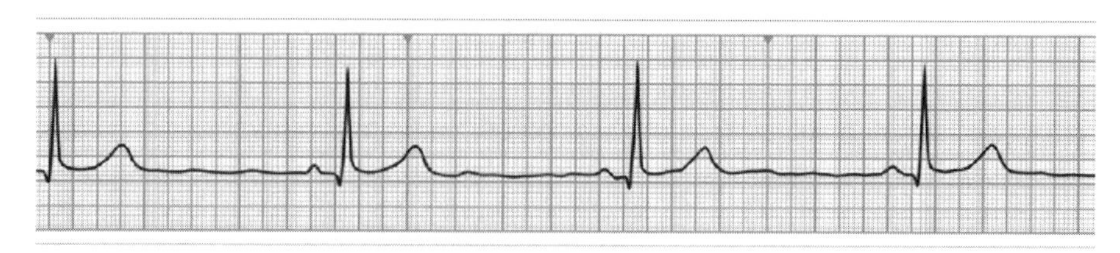

Figure 9.1 Sinus bradycardia. (Reproduced by permission of the Resuscitation Council (UK).)

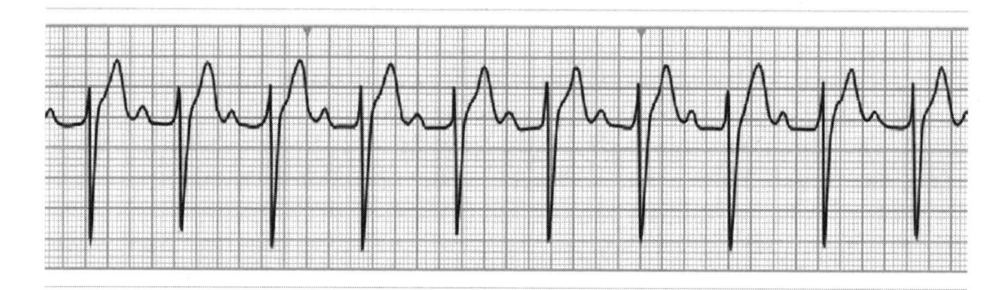

Figure 9.2 First-degree heart block. (Reproduced by permission of the Resuscitation Council (UK).)

and each preceded by a P wave, this looks at first sight like sinus rhythm. The key to this rhythm is that from the start of each P wave to the start of the QRS complexes, the distance is about nine small squares (0.36 seconds). This is prolonged and indicates that the patient is in first-degree heart block. This means that conduction from the atria to the ventricles while not being completely blocked off is being delayed, generally as a result of ischaemia after a myocardial infarction (MI) (Solodky et al. 1998), or in an elderly person as a result of degenerative fibrotic changes of the conduction system (Bharati et al. 1992). First-degree heart block may not require treatment, but it may cause the heart to slow problematically and, if seen, it must always be reported and observed because there is a risk that it may develop into higher grades of block.

SECOND-DEGREE HEART BLOCK MOBITZ TYPE I

In Figure 9.3, we can see immediately that the rhythm is irregular, with different spacings between the QRS complexes. We can also see that at times there is a P wave without a following QRS complex. When we look more carefully we can see that, in the beats preceding the P wave without a QRS complex, the distance between the P waves and the QRS gets progressively longer each beat, leading to the P wave with no QRS. This is a type of heart

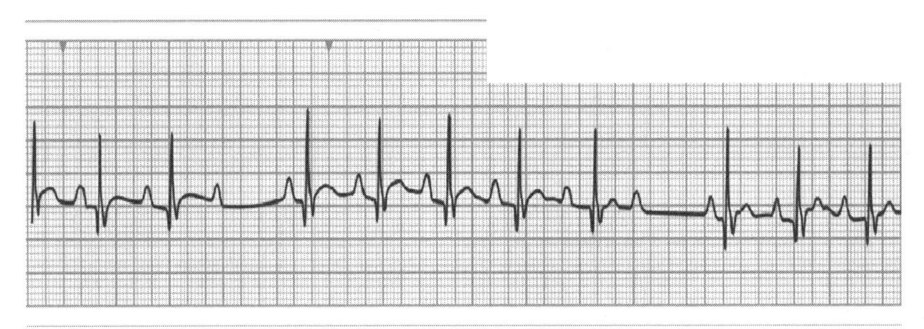

Figure 9.3 Second-degree heart block (Mobitz type I). (Reproduced by permission of the Resuscitation Council (UK).)

block known as second-degree heart block Mobitz type I, which is also often called the Wenckebach phenomenon. We can see the heart rate is varying from about 75 bpm down to about 40 bpm. This is characteristic of this heart rhythm, demonstrating a conduction delay that is gradually increasing until it becomes blocked off completely, before the pattern goes on to repeat itself. If we were watching a continuous recording we would probably see that there were the same number of complexes each time before the missing QRS complex. This has led some people to call it a 'regularly irregular' rhythm, although it is probably easier (and more elegant) to say that it has a cyclical pattern.

Despite its odd appearance, second-degree heart block type I does not often require treatment. There is some evidence that it is quite common in people without producing symptoms and it is more common in elderly people (Andrea et al. 2002).

SECOND-DEGREE HEART BLOCK MOBITZ TYPE II

In Figure 9.4 we can see that the rhythm is regular, with a rate of 27 bpm. Each QRS complex is preceded by a P wave that is associated with it, as we would expect, but in addition there are other P waves present that are not followed by QRS complexes. These features indicate that the rhythm is second-degree heart block Mobitz type II. This indicates that the blocking of the impulses between the atria and the ventricles is now severe, with every second impulse not being conducted. Sometimes the degree of blocking is less severe, with only every third or fourth impulse not getting through. Sometimes this rhythm is called 'two-to-one heart block' (or three- or four-to-one, depending on the degree of block), but it is better to give its correct title to avoid confusion and add on the degree of block for accuracy. So, we could call this second-degree heart block Mobitz type II with a two-to-one block. This rhythm, particularly with a rate as slow as this one, is highly likely to need intervention because the patient is likely to be symptomatic. This rhythm may be found in elderly

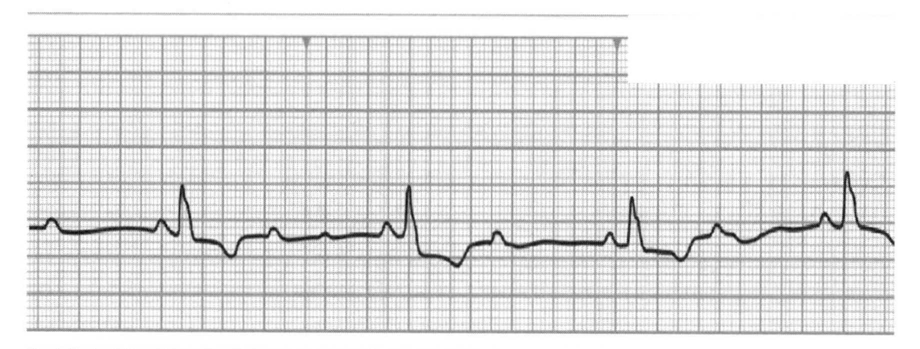

Figure 9.4 Second-degree heart block (Mobitz type II). (Reproduced by permission of the Resuscitation Council (UK).)

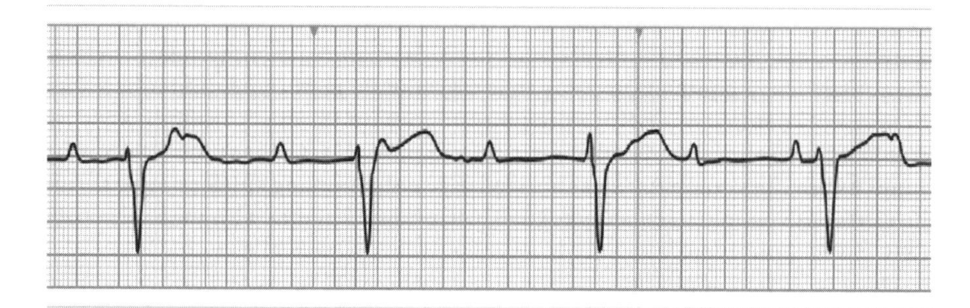

Figure 9.5 Third-degree heart block. (Reproduced by permission of the Resuscitation Council (UK).)

people, but more problematically may be seen acutely after an MI (Altun et al. 1998). Interestingly, the QRS complex is quite broad looking here, indicating that there may be some conduction delay across the ventricles as well.

THIRD-DEGREE HEART BLOCK

In Figure 9.5, the rhythm is regular and has a rate of about 29 bpm. We can see that there are P waves, but none of them seems to be associated with the QRS complexes, which are obviously broad, up to almost five small squares (0.2 seconds) at the widest point. If we were to measure the distance between consecutive P waves, I think that we would find that it was constant assuming, from the different shapes of the T wave in the first and fourth complex and in the start of the QRS of the third complex, that there are buried P waves that we cannot see properly. This indicates that the P waves and the QRS

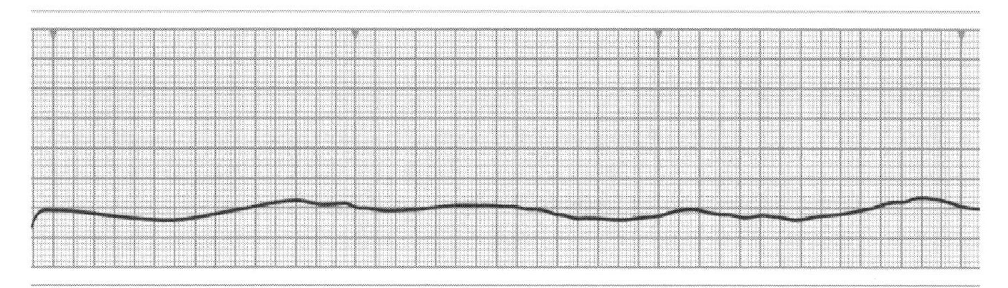

Figure 9.6 Asystole. (Reproduced by permission of the Resuscitation Council (UK).)

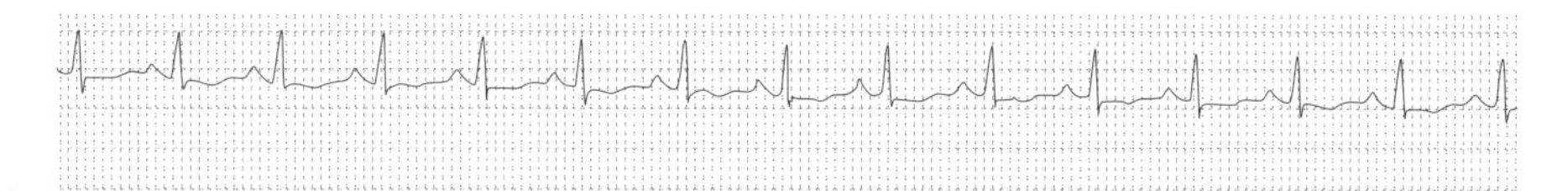

Figure 9.7 Sinus tachycardia.

complexes are both regular but not associated with each other at all. This is third-degree heart block, also called complete heart block. This can be a very problematic condition when associated with an MI, with mortality levels three times higher than for those without this condition (Abidov et al. 2004) and normally needs immediate intervention.

ASYSTOLE

The tracing in Figure 9.6, showing no electrical activity away from the gently undulating baseline, is asystole. Complete heart block may degenerate to this or it may result from other factors such as anoxia. Occasionally P waves may be seen alone. This is always a cardiac arrest rhythm.

EXAMPLES OF TACHYARRHYTHMIAS

SINUS TACHYCARDIA

Figure 9.7 demonstrates a regular rhythm with a heart rate of 115 bpm. The QRS complexes are narrow, which is a good indicator that conduction of the impulse has begun above the ventricle. Although the rhythm is fast, P waves can be seen before each QRS complex. This all adds up to a sinus tachycardia, which is a normal response to sympathetic stimulation of the heart (Klabunde 2005b) if someone is excited, anxious or undergoing some form of exercise, but may also be a sign of an underlying pathophysiological problem such as bleeding (Gupta and Fahim 2005) or thyrotoxicosis (Roffi et al. 2005).

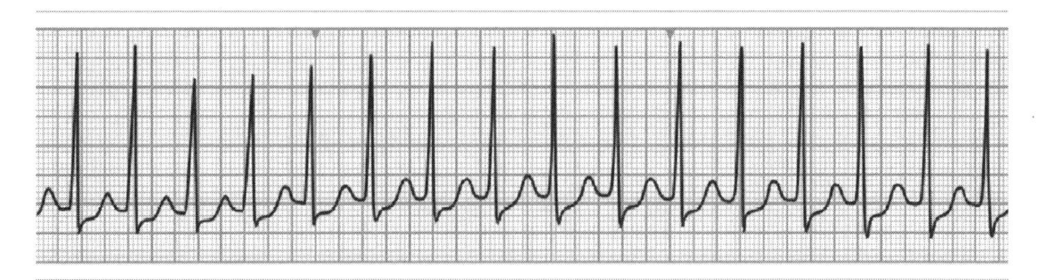

Figure 9.8 Narrow complex tachycardia. (Reproduced by permission of the Resuscitation Council (UK).)

In such circumstances the correct treatment is to manage the underlying condition. Sinus tachycardia can be a classic example of the dictum of the cardiologist who said: 'this patient has an arrhythmia because he is ill, he is not ill because he has an arrhythmia!' (John Caplin 1989, personal communication).

SUPRAVENTRICULAR TACHYCARDIA

In Figure 9.8 we see a regular rhythm with a fast heart rate of about 115 bpm. The QRS complexes are narrow, indicating that the impulse was initiated above the ventricles. The difficulty here is in deciding if there are P waves. I do not think that there are. Generally speaking, T waves are more likely to be present than P waves if, as here, you have one or the other but not both. This means that it is likely that the impulse has come from above the ventricles but not from the SA node. In this circumstance it may be that the impulses have arisen from the AV node, but similar tracings, sometimes with small pointy looking P waves, can come from tachycardias arising in the atria away from the SA node. It is convenient to group tachycardias of this nature together under the heading narrow complex tachycardias (NCTs) or supraventricular tachycardias (SVTs). Either term is acceptable for these rhythms, which are sometimes problematic but rarely life threatening. They can be caused by ischaemia and degeneration, but are more often the result of anatomical irregularities causing re-entry (Roberts-Thomson et al. 2005).

ATRIAL FIBRILLATION

This interesting tracing shows narrow QRS complexes with no obvious P waves, just a lot of bizarre-looking activity between them. The heart rate varies from below 60 bpm at one point to up to 180 bpm, with variations in between. Given that it does seem fast, we could call it a narrow complex tachycardia, but the fact that it is extremely irregular allows us to be more precise here. This is atrial fibrillation, where the atria that are vibrating rather than con-

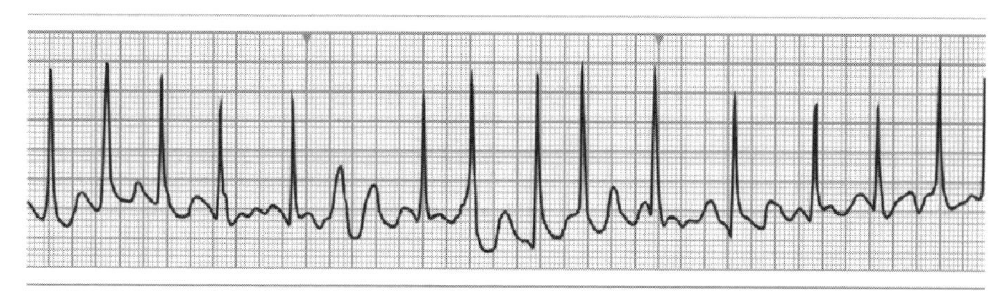

Figure 9.9 Atrial fibrillation. (Reproduced by permission of the Resuscitation Council (UK).)

tracting are producing a lot of electrical activity, resulting in the bizarre waveforms between the QRS complexes. Not all of these impulses conduct through to the ventricles, which respond sporadically, producing the irregular rate of the QRS complexes. The same people who call the Wenckebach phenomenon 'regularly irregular' are likely to call this 'irregularly irregular' but this seems unnecessarily complicating as well as hard to say, so let us just stick with irregular, as it obviously is.

Atrial fibrillation can be caused by structural problems such as mitral valve problems or heart failure but it may be difficult to isolate a cause (Nattel and Opie 2006). It is increasingly recognised as a problematic arrhythmia; as well as being extremely common (particularly among elderly people) and affecting around 1% of the population of the UK as a whole, it is often associated with strokes from clots forming in the blood pooling in the non-contracting left atrium that then migrate to the brain (Stuart et al. 2004).

VENTRICULAR TACHYCARDIA

Figure 9.10 shows broad QRS complexes (up to five small squares – 0.2 seconds) and not much else. It is regular and very fast with a rate of about 215 bpm and no P waves to be seen. The broad QRS complexes are strong pointers to a rhythm arising in the ventricles so, although we can quite correctly call this a broad complex tachycardia, it is highly likely that we can be more precise and call it a ventricular tachycardia (VT). VT can look different to this – it may be irregular and unconnected P waves may be seen – but it is always fast and always broad. VT is extremely problematic and may be sufficiently fast that the ventricles do not have time to fill adequately. The drop in cardiac output can be so severe that cardiac arrest is induced and sudden cardiac death results. VT may be caused by ischaemia or electrolyte imbalance or by a congenital problem such as Brugada's syndrome, among many other possibilities (Stahmer and Cowan 2006). Even if it is not pulseless, it needs treating effectively as a matter of urgency.

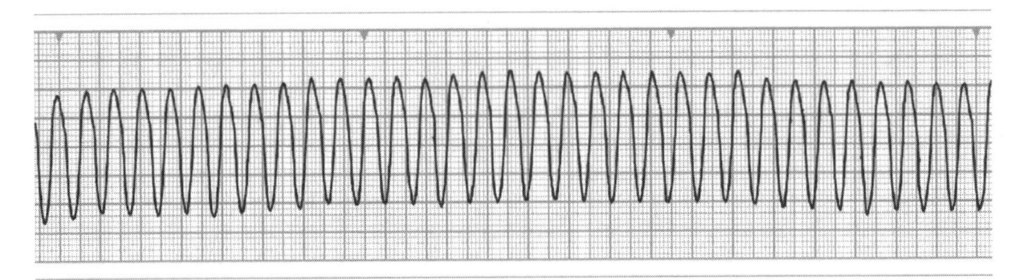

Figure 9.10 Broad complex tachycardia. (Reproduced by permission of the Resuscitation Council (UK).)

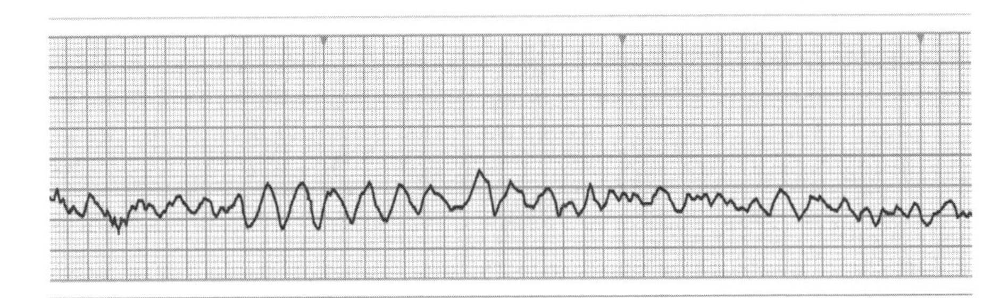

Figure 9.11 Ventricular fibrillation. (Reproduced by permission of the Resuscitation Council (UK).)

VENTRICULAR FIBRILLATION

The bizarre, broad pattern of Figure 9.11 indicates ventricular fibrillation (VF). VF is always a cardiac arrest rhythm.

TREATING BRADYARRHYTHMIAS

In this section I focus on treatment as recommended in the newest version of the Resuscitation Council (UK) guidelines (Figure 9.12). Whether a heart rhythm is fast or slow, it is important to decide whether or not the patient is stable. The haemodynamic consequences of any heart rhythm may vary, and the individual's response will determine whether or not an arrhythmia is going to be problematic.

Adverse signs that may indicate instability are a systolic blood pressure below 90 mmHg, a heart rate below 40 bpm, ventricular ectopic beats and breathlessness indicating heart failure (Resuscitation Council (UK) 2005). If these are detected the patient should be immediately attached to a heart

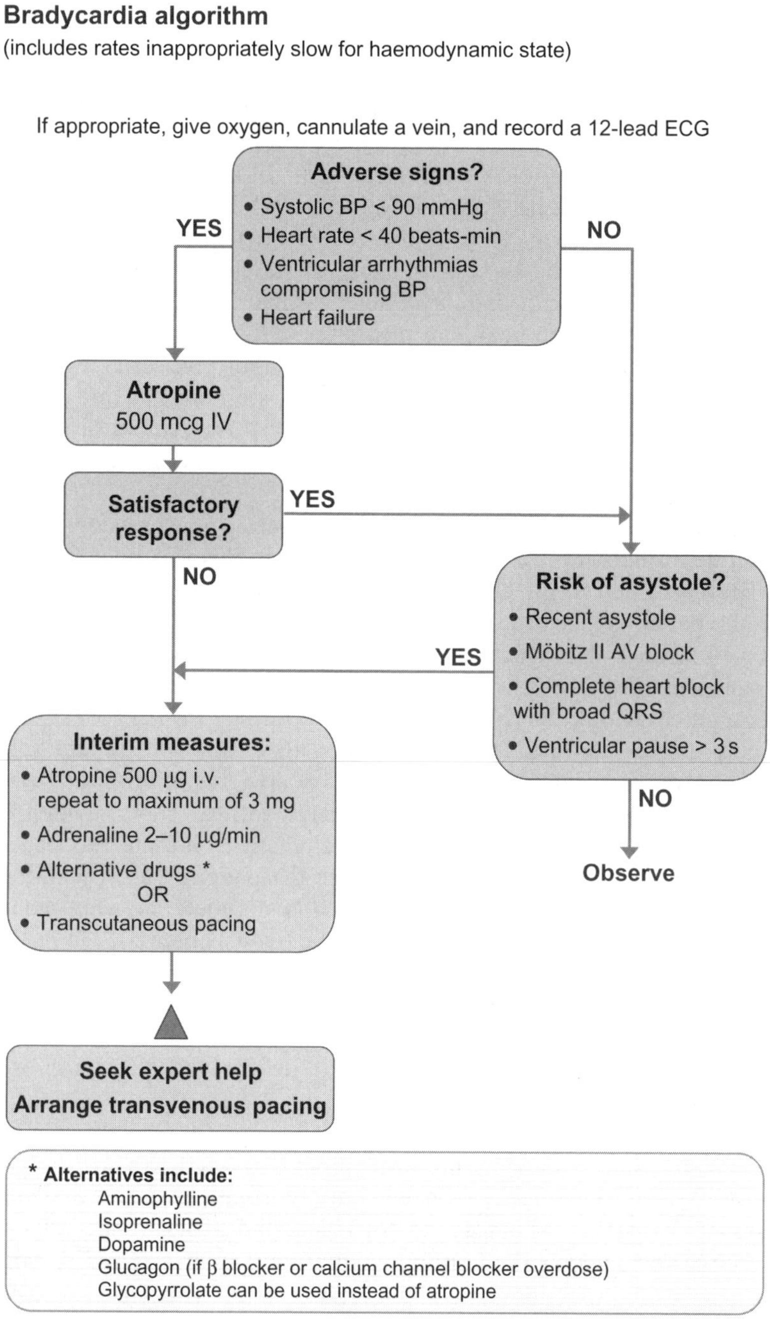

Bradycardia algorithm

(includes rates inappropriately slow for haemodynamic state)

If appropriate, give oxygen, cannulate a vein, and record a 12-lead ECG

Adverse signs?
- Systolic BP < 90 mmHg
- Heart rate < 40 beats-min
- Ventricular arrhythmias compromising BP
- Heart failure

YES → **Atropine** 500 mcg IV → **Satisfactory response?**

NO (adverse signs) → **Risk of asystole?**

Satisfactory response? YES → **Risk of asystole?**

Satisfactory response? NO → **Interim measures**

Risk of asystole?
- Recent asystole
- Möbitz II AV block
- Complete heart block with broad QRS
- Ventricular pause > 3 s

YES → **Interim measures**

NO → **Observe**

Interim measures:
- Atropine 500 μg i.v. repeat to maximum of 3 mg
- Adrenaline 2–10 μg/min
- Alternative drugs *

OR

- Transcutaneous pacing

→ **Seek expert help**
Arrange transvenous pacing

*** Alternatives include:**
Aminophylline
Isoprenaline
Dopamine
Glucagon (if β blocker or calcium channel blocker overdose)
Glycopyrrolate can be used instead of atropine

Figure 9.12 Algorithm for the management of bradyarrhythmias. (Reproduced by permission of the Resuscitation Council (UK).)

monitor and given high-flow oxygen, and venous access should be established and expert help sought.

In the presence of adverse signs, atropine 500 μg should be given intravenously up to a maximum of 3 mg. If this works effectively, the health practitioner should then determine whether there is a risk of asystole, indicated by a recent episode of asystole or complete heart block, especially if the heart rate is below 40 bpm (Resuscitation Council (UK) 2005). If this risk is apparent, or if there has been no response to the atropine, as may be the case (Wesley et al. 1986), the patient is likely to require some form of cardiac pacing. If electrical pacing is unavailable, cardiac fist pacing may be useful (Tucker et al. 1995). The health professional should explain carefully to the patient what she or he intends to do and why and then give serial regular blows with the closed fist over the left lower edge of the sternum, at a rate of between 50 and 70 bpm (Resuscitation Council (UK) 2005). The patient should, where possible, have the pulse palpated so that it can be established that a viable cardiac output is being produced.

Transcutaneous pacing is a useful and perhaps underused option. Many modern defibrillators have the capacity to pace in this way once pacing pads have been attached to the chest wall of the patient. The pacemaker will then sense the patient's heart rate and deliver external electrical pulses across the chest wall through the myocardium to stimulate contraction. Operation of the pacemaker/defibrillator is not difficult and health professionals with access to this equipment should be routinely trained to initiate this. These pacemakers routinely deliver 'demand' pacing, meaning that they will initiate a pacing impulse only if they detect that the patient's heart rate has dropped below the rate at which the transcutaneous pacemaker is set. Anecdotal evidence suggests that some health professionals are reluctant to initiate this procedure because of the discomfort that it may cause the patient. This discomfort can be minimised by careful explanation of what is intended and what the consequences will be, along with a reiteration of the likely benefits. If the procedure is painful to the patient, this can be minimised by appropriate use of analgesia and sedation, and by ensuring that the pacing is performed at the lowest possible effective electrical current (Gould and Marshall 1988). It may also help to remember the discomfort and risk of death to the patient if an intervention is delayed or not attempted.

Both fist pacing and transcutaneous pacing are essentially emergency options as a result of their nature and the risk of discomfort to the patient. The gold standard emergency management of atropine-resistant bradycardias is transvenous pacing, where a catheter is inserted under a local anaesthetic into a large vein such as the femoral or internal jugular, and fed through the caval opening and right atrium into the right ventricle. The part of the catheter external to the patient is then attached to a pacemaker system that can be regulated to pace the heart at a given rate, usually in the demand mode. This is more stable than transcutaneous pacing and is essentially the same technology involved in permanent pacing, where a self-contained pacemaker is attached as described with the pulse generator element inserted subcutaneously. Permanent pacing may be required for persistent bradyarrhythmias, particularly in elderly people. More information about temporary and permanent pacing can be found in Chapter 14.

TREATING TACHYARRHYTHMIAS

Again, the initial emphasis should be on treating adverse signs, which may include chest pain, and in establishing cardiac monitoring, high-flow oxygen and venous access, and seeking expert help (Figure 9.13). The standard treatment for unstable tachyarrhythmias is to attempt DC cardioversion. This is an attempt to shock the heart into a more viable rhythm by re-establishing the SA node as the dominant pacemaker. It is the same principle as defibrillation, except that the shock device is synchronised, by means of its monitoring facility, to deliver the shock precisely on the R wave of the QRS complex. This avoids the vulnerable period of cardiac repolarisation, which corresponds to the T wave on the ECG. Synchronised cardioversion can normally be delivered at a lower energy setting than is used for defibrillation. As patients are often conscious in this circumstance, it is essential that they be sedated or anaesthetised before the procedure is attempted. If cardioversion is unsuccessful on up to three shocks, then amiodarone 300 mg i.v. should be given over 10–20 minutes, followed by a further shock attempt and an infusion of amiodarone 900 mg over 24 hours (Resuscitation Council (UK) 2005).

If the patient is stable, this gives more opportunity to assess the rhythm, and the crucial decision is whether the tachycardia is broad or narrow complex. If it is broad and regular, amiodarone can be given over 24 hours. If it is irregular, this may be more problematic. Electrolyte abnormality, particularly low potassium levels, should be corrected as a first priority, and magnesium sulphate 2 mg should be given over 10 minutes (Resuscitation Council (UK) 2005). There is a high chance of such a rhythm predisposing to adverse features, in which case synchronised cardioversion should be rapidly arranged, or of it becoming pulseless, so careful monitoring of the patient is imperative.

NCTs without adverse signs may be treated with vagal manoeuvres. These are attempts to stimulate the vagus nerve because this has a considerable 'braking' effect on the heart, by activating the PNS. The cells responsive to such stimulus are predominantly situated in the AV node and are least likely to be present in the ventricles, so these manoeuvres are indicated in NCTs only as the impulses have been initiated above the ventricles. Vagal measures include the Valsalva manoeuvre, where a patient can be encouraged to attempt to blow the plunger of a syringe out of the barrel, sucking ice or drinking cold fluids (ideally small sips in case synchronised cardioversion with anaesthetisation is later required) or plunging the face into cold water. Carotid sinus

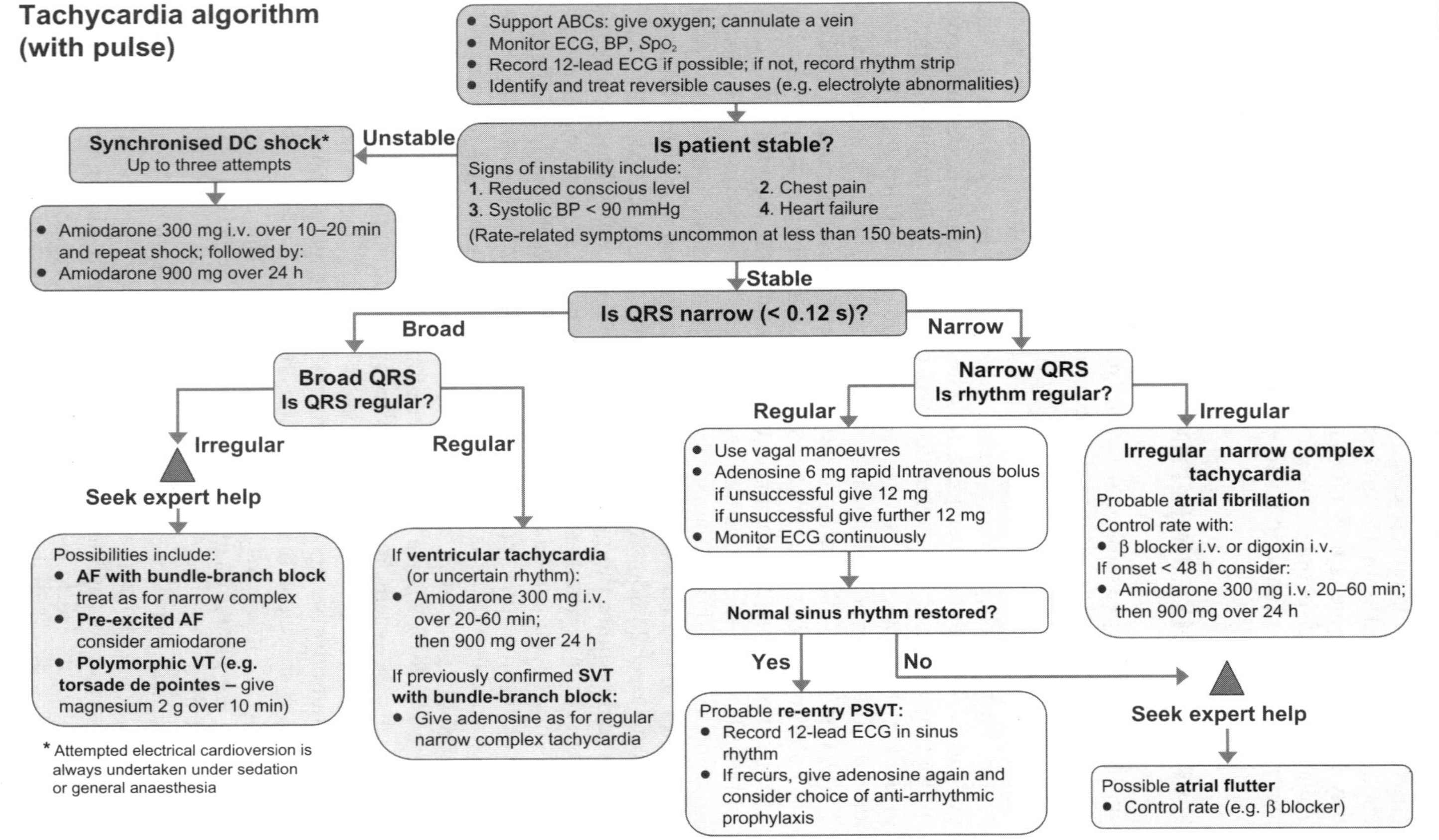

Figure 9.13 Algorithm for the management of tachyarrhythmias. (Reproduced by permission of the Resuscitation Council (UK).)

massage is a very effective vagal manoeuvre, but it is contraindicated in the presence of carotid bruits, and these should be checked for by a specialist before this is attempted, because there is a risk of a stroke from a dislodged atheromatous plaque in this circumstance. If no bruits are present carotid sinus massage is a safe procedure (Richardson et al. 2000). If there is no response to this, adenosine 6 mg should be given. If this is ineffective, 12 mg should be given, followed by a further 12 mg if there is still no result. Vagal manoeuvres will terminate most regular NCTs. If they do not, verapamil given intravenously is an option that may be tried (Resuscitation Council (UK) 2005).

Irregular NCTs are very likely to be AF and so carry the additional risk of clot formation, particularly if the patient is believed to have been in the rhythm for longer than 48 hours. If this is thought to be the case, the patient should ideally be fully anticoagulated for at least 3 weeks, if in a sufficiently stable haemodynamic state. If the rate needs to be controlled, rate-controlling drugs such as β blockers, digoxin or magnesium may be considered as an alternative to electrical cardioversion or chemical cardioversion with amiodarone. If the duration is less than 48 hours, cardioversion may be an option (Resuscitation Council (UK) 2005).

In the long term, potentially lethal arrhythmias are now being managed with implanted cardiac defibrillators (ICDs) which have the ability to pace the heart very rapidly and then slow it down once they have 'captured' the heart rhythm (overdrive or anti-tachycardia pacing); if this fails, they can deliver a low-energy shock directly to the heart. These devices undoubtedly save lives but have been shown to be associated with a high level of anxiety in those in whom they are implanted (Hegel et al. 2000). ICD implantation is discussed in more detail in Chapter 14.

CONCLUSION

Cardiac arrhythmias are problematic and potentially lethal. They have a multiplicity of causative factors and mechanisms and can usefully be classified as bradyarrhythmias or tachyarrhythmias. They can best be managed by a systematic approach to cardiac monitoring that will enable the health professional to determine the most effective management. Electrical methods such as cardioversion or pacing are likely to be more effective treatment avenues than drugs and should be tried if the rhythm is unstable, as demonstrated by the presence of adverse signs. Haemodynamic consequences of any given arrhythmia will vary, so it is vital that the patient be treated, not the rhythm.

REFERENCES

Abidov A, Kaluski E, Hod H et al. (2004) Influence of conduction disturbances on clinical outcome in patients with acute myocardial infarction receiving thrombolysis (results from the ARGAMI-2 study). *American Journal of Cardiology* **93**(1): 76–80.

Altun A, Kirdar C, Ozbay G (1998) Effect of aminophylline in patients with atropine-resistant late advanced atrioventricular block during acute inferior myocardial infarction. *Clinical Cardiology* **21**: 759–62.

Andrea E, Atie J, Maciel W et al. (2002) Intra-His bundle block: clinical, electrocardiographic, and electrophysiologic characteristics. *Arquivos Brasileiros de Cardiologia* **79**: 532–7.

Bharati S, Surawicz B, Vidaillet HJ Jr et al. (1992) Familial congenital sinus rhythm anomalies: clinical and pathological correlations. *Pacing and Clinical Electrophysiology* **15**(11 Pt 1): 1720–9.

Da Costa D, Brady WJ, Edhouse J (2002) ABC of clinical electrocardiography: Bradycardias and atrioventricular conduction block. *British Medical Journal* **324**: 535–8.

Department of Health (2005) *National Service Framework for Coronary Heart Disease.* London: HMSO.

Gould B, Marshall A (1988) Noninvasive temporary pacemakers. *Pacing and Clinical Electrophysiology* **11**: 1331–5.

Gupta RK, Fahim M (2005) Regulation of cardiovascular functions during acute blood loss. *Indian Journal of Physiological Pharmacology* **49**: 213–19.

Hegel M, Griegel L, Black C et al. (2000) Anxiety and depression in patients receiving implanted cardioverter-defibrillators: a longitudinal investigation. *International Journal of Psychiatry in Medicine* **27**(1): 57–69.

Jacobson C (2000) Arrhythmias and conduction disturbances. In: Woods S, Froelicher E, Motzer S (eds), *Cardiac Nursing*, 4th edn. Philadelphia: Lippincott, Williams & Wilkins, pp 297–362.

Jensen-Urstad K, Saltin B, Ericson M et al. (1997) Pronounced resting bradycardia in male elite runners is associated with high heart rate variability. *Scandinavian Journal of Medical Science in Sports* **5**: 274–8.

Julian D, Campbell-Cowan J, McLenachan J (2005) *Cardiology*. London: WB Saunders.

Klabunde R (2005a) *Overdrive Suppression.* Available from www.cvphysiology.com/Arrhythmias/A018.htm

Klabunde RE (2005b) *Autonomic Innervation of the Heart and Vasculature*. Available from www.cvphysiology.com/Blood%20Pressure/BP008.htm

Nattel S, Opie LH (2006) Controversies in atrial fibrillation. *Lancet* **367**: 262–72.

Resuscitation Council (UK) (2000) *Advanced Life Support Manual*. London: Resuscitation Council (UK).

Resuscitation Council (UK) (2005) *Resuscitation Council Guidelines 2005*. London: Resuscitation Council (UK).

Richardson D, Bexton R, Shaw F et al. (2000) Complications of carotid sinus massage – a prospective series of older patients. *Age and Aging* **29**: 413–17.

Roberts-Thomson K, Kistler P, Kalman J (2005) Atrial tachycardia: mechanisms, diagnosis, and management. *Current problems in Cardiology* **30**: 529–73.

Roffi M, Cattaneo F, Brandle M (2005) Thyrotoxicosis and the cardiovascular system. *Minerva Endocrinology* **30**(2): 47–58.

Smith J, Kampine J (1990) *Circulatory Physiology*, 3rd edn. Baltimore, MD: Williams & Wilkins.

Solodky A, Assali A, Herz I et al. (1998) Early development of high-degree atrioventricular block in inferior acute myocardial infarction is predicted by a J-point/R-wave ratio above 0.5 on admission. *Cardiology* **90**: 274–9.

Stahmer SA, Cowan R (2006) Tachydysrhythmias. *Emergency Medical Clinic of North America* **24**(1): 11–40, v–vi.

Stuart S, Murphy N, Walker A et al. (2004) Cost of an emerging epidemic: an economic analysis of atrial fibrillation in the UK. *Heart* **90**: 286–92.

Tucker KJ, Shaburihvili TS, Gedevanishvili A (1995) Manual external (fist) pacing during high-degree atrioventricular block: a lifesaving intervention *American Journal of Emergency Medicine* **3**(1): 53–4.

Wesley R Jr, Lerman B, DiMarco J et al. (1986) Mechanism of atropine-resistant atrioventricular block during inferior myocardial infarction: possible role of adenosine. *Journal of American Cardiology* **8**: 1232–4.

10 Resuscitation

JOANNE HATFIELD

Cardiac arrest – the cessation of heart function – is the ultimate medical emergency, leading rapidly to death unless timely and appropriate action (resuscitation) is taken. Respiratory arrest – cessation of breathing – may occur with cardiac arrest ('cardiopulmonary arrest') or with the heart continuing to beat before eventually succumbing to hypoxia. The health professional will encounter an 'arrest' in the clinical setting, commonplace in hospital accident and emergency departments (A&E), cardiac or critical care units (CCUs) or general medical wards, but also on occasion in the setting of the surgical or gynaecological ward, and less often but not unheard of in the outpatient clinic or other department. Most cardiac arrests occur, however, in the community setting, and about three-quarters of these in patients' homes. Ambulance personnel have arguably the greatest exposure to resuscitation practice. The health professional may be called on to start resuscitation as a bystander, neighbour or even relative. Chances of survival after an arrest remain very poor despite advances in science.

The mainstay of resuscitation, closed chest cardiac massage, is a relatively recent phenomenon, having been described in the late twentieth century by Kouwenhoven and Jude (1960). Resuscitation measures should be considered time dependent because the heart and brain do not survive more than a few minutes without adequate oxygenation. Cardiopulmonary resuscitation (CPR) is practised by health professionals and laypeople in and out of the hospital setting. This chapter attempts to summarise current guidelines for resuscitation of adults by health professionals.

CPR comprises two principal activities: basic life support (BLS) and advanced life support (ALS). BLS describes measures to clear the airway and artificially support breathing and circulation without use of equipment (Nolan 1998, Quinn and Hatchett 2002, Jowett and Thompson 2003). BLS aims to maintain a degree of cerebral and coronary perfusion, slowing the rate of cell deterioration until definitive treatment (ALS) can be provided. Spontaneous recovery after BLS alone is rare, so BLS should be considered as a 'holding measure' until appropriate equipment and trained personnel arrive to administer ALS.

Cardiac Care: An Introduction for Healthcare Professionals. Edited by David Barrett, Mark Gretton and Tom Quinn
© 2006 John Wiley & Sons Ltd

ALS involves the use of equipment and drugs to maintain the airway, attempt to correct heart rhythm disturbances and support cardiac function. A new term 'immediate life support' (ILS) is emerging, describing use of simple airway adjuncts and automated defibrillation, which require less intensive training than ALS.

THE CHAIN OF SURVIVAL

The sequences of BLS and ALS techniques are considered together as a 'chain of survival' (Cummins et al. 1991, Resuscitation Council (UK) 2006) made up of the following links:

- Early recognition and call for help: to ensure that appropriate help is summoned as soon as possible.
- Early BLS: to provide oxygen to the heart and brain, buying time pending arrival of trained personnel and equipment.
- Early defibrillation: to restart the heart
- Post-resuscitation care: to support vital functions, and progress recovery towards a good quality of life.

The public, and professional bodies, expect healthcare professionals to be able to react appropriately in an emergency to help save lives. Survival after a witnessed cardiac arrest can be doubled if bystander resuscitation is attempted (Larsen et al. 1993, Waalewijn et al. 2001). ALS techniques should, however, be undertaken only by those competent to do so (Resuscitation Council (UK) 2005). Health professionals should as a minimum be able to perform BLS and undergo annual updates to maintain competence (Gabbott et al. 2005). Training should cover recognising cardiac arrest, getting help, starting BLS (using airway adjuncts) and attempting defibrillation (Gabbott et al. 2005).

IMPORTANCE OF EARLY DEFIBRILLATION

Defibrillation is the key intervention to correct ventricular fibrillation (VF), the chaotic heart rhythm disorder commonly associated with early stages of cardiac arrest. Where the presenting rhythm is ventricular tachycardia (VT) without a pulse, this is treated as VF. The success of defibrillation is largely time dependent: if delivered within 3 minutes, the reported survival rate is almost twice that if delivered later (Peberdy et al. 2003).

Most patients who sustain cardiac arrest die as a result. Survival rates have not appreciably improved despite developments in drug therapy and equipment. Survival to discharge after cardiac arrest in hospital ranges from 6–10%

in patients presenting in asystole or pulseless electrical activity (PEA), and up to 35–42% in VF/VT (Gwinnutt et al. 2000, Peberdy et al. 2003). For out-of-hospital arrests, percentage survival rates are in dismal single figures.

PREVENTION IS BETTER THAN CURE

There is renewed emphasis on early identification of hospitalised patients considered at risk of cardiac arrest. About 80% of patients who arrest will have displayed 'warning' signs such as tachycardia, bradycardia, hypotension, dyspnoea, altered conscious level and poor urine output documented in the hours leading up to the event (Resuscitation Council (UK) 2000). Steps to prevent cardiac arrest may improve outcomes. The use of medical emergency teams (METs) or critical care outreach teams to respond to acute patient crises, identified by risk scores based on the above warning signs (Gabbott et al. 2005), has been associated with a reduction in hospital arrests (Buist et al. 2002). The assessment of a patient at risk of cardiac arrest is explored in greater depth in Chapter 5.

BLS FOR THE HEALTHCARE PROFESSIONAL

Equipment and personnel are more readily available in some clinical settings than others. In the community setting, ambulance technicians and paramedics, and some others acting as 'first responders', increasingly have access to much of the equipment and drugs available to the hospital team.

SAFETY FIRST

Safety of the 'rescuer' is paramount. Electrical cables, wet or polished floors, and over-protective pet dogs are just examples of potential hazards (beware, for instance, the full water jug or urinal on the bedside locker!). The risk of infection with HIV, tuberculosis and hepatitis, although low, should always be taken seriously and universal precautions applied. Eye protection and gloves should be worn during resuscitation attempts. Care should be taken to prevent sharps injuries and disposal equipment should be available (Resuscitation Council (UK) 2002). Caution must be taken before moving or attempting to catch a collapsing patient, to avoid injury to the rescuer.

INITIAL ASSESSMENT

Once personal safety had been established, a 'shake-and-shout' approach is recommended to establish the patient's level of responsiveness. If there is no response, the rescuer should shout for help. In hospital, the emergency call button should be activated. In the community, an ambulance should be summoned using the 999 system.

A – airway

The patient's mouth should be checked for any visible obstruction, which should be removed with fingers or suction. If suction is used, the tip of the catheter should be seen at all times (Moule and Albarran 2005). Well-fitting dentures should be left in place as this will help provide a good seal for a facemask; loose dentures place the airway at risk and should be removed (and put somewhere for safe keeping).

A 'head-tilt, chin-lift' manoeuvre should be employed to open the airway. One hand should be placed on the forehead and two fingers under the chin lifting until the teeth almost close: this prevents the tongue falling back and allows air entry into the lungs if the patient is breathing. If there is suspicion of neck injury, use of a jaw thrust should be considered. Kneeling at the head of the casualty, feel with the fingers along the jaw to behind the angle; the balls of the thumbs are placed on the maxilla, lifting anteriorly. The thumbs can be used to open the mouth to enable assessment. This also draws the tongue forward and opens the airway (Chellel 2000, Jevon 2002, Colquhoun et al. 2004).

B and C – breathing and circulation

Simultaneous assessment of breathing and circulation should take no more than 10 seconds. Assess breathing by looking for chest wall movement, listening for normal breathing sounds and feeling for exhaled air on the cheek or palm of the hand. If breathing does not appear normal (e.g. agonal gasping) this should be classed as 'not breathing': if in doubt act as though there is no breathing (Handley et al. 2005). In assessing the circulation, even experienced personnel have difficulty locating the carotid pulse (Bahr et al. 1997): using the index and middle finger, tracing down the trachea to the larynx, slide the fingers into the hollow of the neck (either side will do). Observing the patient for movement, coughing or breathing can more readily assess adequacy of circulation (Perkins et al. 2005). The findings of this initial assessment will guide the rescuer to the intervention required as discussed below.

BLS INTERVENTIONS

If both breathing and pulse detected

The unconscious patient will benefit from being placed in the recovery position to help maintain a patent airway, allowing the tongue to fall forwards and gastric contents or saliva to drain from the mouth.

If pulse detected but no breathing

This is respiratory arrest and requires assisted ventilation at a rate of 10 breaths/min, using available equipment (in the clinical environment equipment such as pocket masks and bag–valve mask devices should be readily to hand), with supplementary oxygen as soon as it is available. Each assisted breath should last one second and produce a chest rise as seen in normal breathing. If help has not already been summoned it should be called for after 1 minute (dial 2222 in hospital or 999 in the community). The patient should be reassessed every minute (especially for signs of circulation).

If no breathing, and no pulse

A call for help using 2222 or 999 is required immediately. A precordial thump with the side of a clenched fist, from a height of 20 cm, to the patient's sternum may be administered if defibrillation is not readily available. If delivered promptly, the thump may be successful at terminating the cardiac arrest rhythm (11–25% chance of success if VT and 2% chance if VF) (Kerber and Robertson 1996). In the absence of circulation, BLS should be commenced without delay: 30 chest compressions should be performed at a rate of 100/minute (just less than two per second), and should precede rescue breathing. The heel of the rescuer's hand should be placed on the middle of the lower half of the sternum in the centre of the chest (Handley 2002), putting the other hand on top and interlocking the fingers. Pressure should not be applied to any other part of the chest wall. The rescuer should use their body weight to push down on the patient's chest to a depth of 4–5 cm, releasing the pressure by letting the hands come up with the chest wall. Hands should remain on the chest wall, while still allowing the chest to recoil fully. Once the 30 compressions have been performed, open the airway and attempt two breaths.

It is extremely important to minimise 'time off chest' so that adequate coronary perfusion pressures are maintained and chances of survival improved: once breaths have been delivered, return immediately to chest compressions. The rate and ratio of chest compressions to rescue breaths (30:2) is the same irrespective of whether there are one or two rescuers. The rate and depth of compressions should be maintained throughout the resuscitation attempt. Chest compressions are tiring and as soon as help is available roles should be changed every 2 min (Handley et al. 2005), ensuring that this is done as smoothly as possible.

Compression-only CPR acceptable

There may be reluctance, in the absence of equipment, to perform mouth-to-mouth ventilation. In such circumstances it is now considered acceptable to administer chest compressions only during the initial stages of a resuscitation attempt. Chest compressions alone may be as effective as compressions and ventilation (Berg et al. 2000). Ventilation should be commenced as soon as the appropriate equipment arrives. BLS should continue without stopping for reassessment until told to stop by qualified personnel or until the patient shows signs of life.

ADVANCED LIFE SUPPORT

Early arrival of ALS trained personnel may be crucial to improving the patient's chances of survival. The Resuscitation Council (UK) (2005) guidelines are summarised in Figure 10.1. BLS is incorporated in the first part of the algorithm, followed by guidance on ALS measures.

The patient's electrocardiogram (ECG) rhythm should be monitored as soon as equipment (ideally a monitor defibrillator) is available. This facilitates decision-making about further treatment as set out in Figure 10.1. It is important to confirm which ECG lead is being monitored, because some defibrillators default to ECG lead II whereas in other cases paddle monitoring is the default lead, resulting in different information being displayed on the monitor. With manual defibrillators, ECG monitoring is rapidly achieved by placing the defibrillator paddles on the patient's chest. Health professionals would be expected to have a working knowledge of the resuscitation equipment in their clinical area.

PULSELESS VT/VF: SHOCKABLE RHYTHMS

As indicated in Figure 10.1 patients in pulseless VT/VF require defibrillation (see below). In the community setting, if the cardiac arrest is not witnessed by a health professional, attempted defibrillation should be preceded by 2 minutes of BLS to improve the chances of success. In hospital, defibrillation should not be delayed.

'Biphasic' defibrillators are widely available and require lower energy delivery to the myocardium than conventional 'monophasic' equipment. A biphasic defibrillator delivers its energy to the myocardium in a positive direction for a specified amount of time and then in a negative direction for the remainder of the time. Underlying physiological mechanisms of biphasic defibrillators are not yet fully understood.

Current guidelines (Resuscitation Council (UK) 2005) advocate defibrillation delivered as single shocks interspersed by BLS, in contrast to previous advice to deliver 'stacks' of three shocks. The evidence base for either strategy is weak, although it has been demonstrated that the effectiveness of the first shock with biphasic defibrillators exceeds 90% (Resuscitation Council (UK) 2005). The new recommendation is predicated in part on observations that the number and quality of chest compressions administered during resuscitation are suboptimal: every effort should be made to continue chest compressions.

Adult advanced life support algorithm

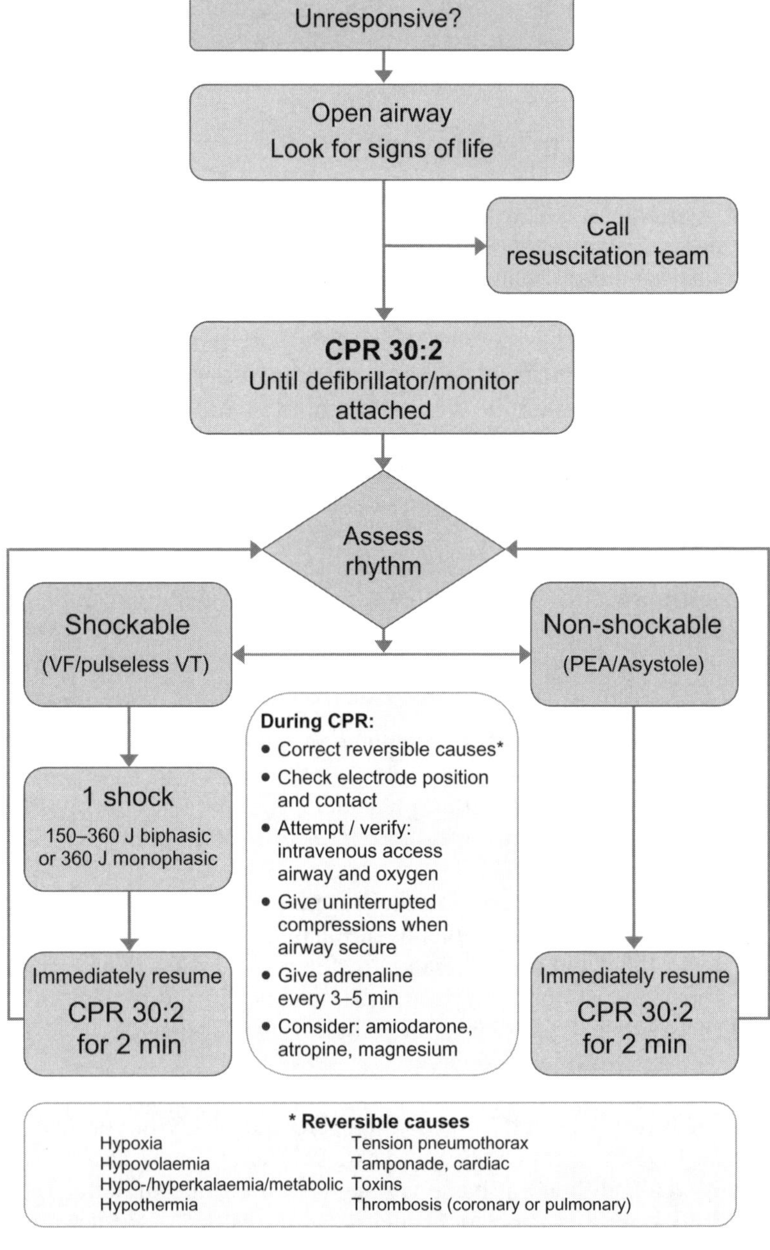

Figure 10.1 Advanced life support algorithm. (Reproduced by permission of the Resuscitation Council (UK).)

Defibrillation

The aim of defibrillation is to deliver energy to the myocardium, interrupting the chaotic heart rhythm (pulseless VT/VF) and allowing the normal conduction system to take over (Resuscitation Council (UK) 2000, Moule and Albarran 2005). Defibrillation can be delivered either manually (by ALS-trained personnel) or via automated external defibrillators (AEDs), the latter being increasingly available in both hospital and community settings such as rail stations and airports (Davies et al. 2005) for use by minimally trained responders.

Safety is a key consideration when using a defibrillator. The patient's chest should be clear of fluids, jewellery, ECG electrodes, wires and patches (e.g. nitrates) to reduce the risk of burns or electrical arcing. When the chest is clear, gel pads (increasingly, self-adhesive electrodes) are placed on the chest to the right of the sternum under the clavicle and to the left of the chest in the area of ECG lead positions V5 and V6 (sternum/apex position). Oxygen flow is a fire hazard and connecting tubes should be removed to at least one metre before shock delivery (Resuscitation Council (UK) 2005). If the patient has a permanent pacemaker *in situ*, care should be taken to place defibrillator paddles/pads 12–15 cm away from the site (Resuscitation Council (UK) 2000). Newer pacemakers are insulated and may withstand defibrillation. A specialist cardiac physiologist should be asked to check the pacing system after successful defibrillation. If using a manual defibrillator, around 8 kg pressure should be applied through the paddles to the chest to reduce transthoracic impedance and increase chances of shock success.

Before shock delivery, it is important to undertake a visual check of the immediate area and shout a firm 'Stand clear!' warning to other resuscitation team members/bystanders, and to make a final confirmation (where appropriate) of the ECG rhythm. It is the ultimate responsibility of the person who presses the 'shock' button to ensure that it is safe to do so.

NON VT/VF: 'NON-SHOCKABLE' RHYTHMS

The 'non-shockable' ECG rhythms in cardiac arrest are asystole and Pulseless Electrical Activity (PEA). In asystole, no electrical activity is evident on the ECG, the monitor picture often being described as a sea swell or undulating baseline. PEA refers to absence of a pulse in the presence of an ECG rhythm normally associated with a palpable pulse.

When treating non-shockable rhythms, priority is given to chest compressions with BLS performed in 2-minute cycles. Every 2 minutes the ECG rhythm and pulse are reassessed; BLS continues if there has been no change in the patient's condition. Airway management depends on available skills. Feasibility of use of a laryngeal mask airway (LMA) by nurses, paramedics and medical staff has been demonstrated. Intubation with an endotracheal

(ET) tube remains the gold standard (Grayling et al. 2002). If an ET tube is inserted, the 30:2 chest compressions:breaths ratio is modified so that continuous chest compressions are administered, with 10 breaths being delivered/minute, without the need to synchronise these activities. When intravenous or intraosseous (I/O) access for administration is unobtainable, some resuscitation drugs (notably adrenaline) can be administered down the ET tube, although rate of absorption is unclear and increased dosages will be required.

In reality many interventions take place simultaneously during a resuscitation attempt. If not already available, intravenous access should be attempted; peripheral cannulation may be the easiest option, although central access is preferable if appropriate skills are available.

DRUGS DURING RESUSCITATION

- Adrenaline 1mg (1 in 10000) should be given every 3–5 minutes (every other cycle of 30 compressions:2 ventilations) to improve cerebral and myocardial perfusion followed by a 20ml flush of physiological or 0.9% saline. The first dose of adrenaline is given as soon as IV access is available in non-shockable rhythms, and prior to the 3rd shock in shockable rhythms. Adrenaline is the only drug that is common to both sides (shockable and non-shockable) of the algorithm.
- Amiodarone 300mg is an anti-arrhythmic drug, and is given for persistent VT/VF, before delivery of the fourth shock. Ideally amiodarone should be given into a large central vein but, in the resuscitation setting, it is considered acceptable to be given (with caution) into a peripheral vein.
- Up to 3mg atropine can be given in PEA when the heart rate is below 60 beats per minute, or in asystole. There is no evidence that atropine improves survival (Engdahl et al. 2001).

PACING

Although temporary transcutaneous (external) or transvenous pacing is unlikely to be of benefit in true asystole (Colquhoun et al. 2004), it may be helpful in the treatment of ventricular standstill or profound bradycardia. The ECG should be checked carefully for any P waves without ventricular activity, or a slow ventricular rhythm that may respond to pacing (Resuscitation Council (UK) 2005).

POTENTIALLY REVERSIBLE CAUSES: 4HS, 4TS

While resuscitation is continuing, the leader of the cardiac arrest team should consider possible reversible causes of the arrest irrespective of the ECG rhythm. The main reversible causes – summarised as the 4Hs and 4Ts – are discussed below.

Hypoxia

This is a reduction in the amount of oxygen supplied to body tissue, and can be assessed by confirming that the patient's airway is clear and lungs are being inflated adequately by artificial ventilation, and that supplementary oxygen is being delivered at the highest concentration. Can bilateral air entry be heard? Is the ET tube in the correct position?

Hypothermia

This is classified as mild (32–35°C), moderate (30–32°C) or severe (<30°C). What is the patient's temperature? Hypothermia should be suspected if the patient has been rescued from water or has been found collapsed in a cold environment. Attempts should be made to warm the patient using appropriate active and passive, internal and external methods. BLS should be continued throughout re-warming, and resuscitation attempts in hypothermic patients may be extremely lengthy.

Hypovolaemia

This is a decreased volume of circulating blood. It may be identified by a history of recent surgery or trauma, suspected ectopic pregnancy or use of anticoagulants (for example). The ECG may show PEA. Circulatory volume should be replaced rapidly with fluids while CPR continues. Expert help should be sought quickly to evaluate further and take appropriate action to stem any bleeding.

Hyper-/hypokalaemia and metabolic disorders

The patient's history (e.g. renal failure, diabetic ketoacidosis) may help; confirmation should be sought by sending blood for urea and electrolyte estimation and arterial blood gas analysis. Potassium levels >5.0 mmol/l may profoundly affect the myocardium. Calcium chloride 10% (10 ml) may be required intravenously. Sodium bicarbonate may be used to treat hyperkalaemia and overdose of a tricyclic antidepressant. If the potassium is too low (hypokalaemia, <3.5 mmol/l) there is a risk of ventricular arrhythmia and potassium infusion may be required. Cardiac arrests caused by hypocalcaemia are rare: the history might reveal muscle tightening, tetany and prolonged QT on the ECG. Treatment is slow intravenous injection of calcium chloride 10%.

Tension pneumothorax

This is when air leaks out of the lung into the interpleural space. The lung collapses, interrupting venous return to the heart, and causing PEA. There may be a history of asthma, recent chest trauma or central line insertion. Signs of

Table 10.1 Drugs and antidotes

Drug	Antidote
Paracetamol	*N*-Acetylcysteine
Organophosphates	Atropine (high dose)
Cyanide	Sodium nitrate
Benzodiazepines	Flumazenil
Opioids	Naloxone
Tricyclic antidepressants	Sodium bicarbonate
β Blockers	Glucagon

From Resuscitation Council (UK) (2000).

a tension pneumothorax include reduced air entry to the affected side, enlarged neck veins, hyperresonance of the affected side and tracheal deviation. Immediate treatment is needle decompression by a wide-bore venous cannula.

Tamponade

Build-up of fluid or blood in the pericardial sac squeezes the heart, which is then unable to fill adequately, potentially causing PEA. Blood/fluid is removed by needle pericardiocentesis.

Toxic/therapeutic disorders

Poisoning (deliberate or accidental) is the primary cause of death under the age of 40 (Resuscitation Council (UK) 2000). Cardiac arrest may be secondary to respiratory failure. If the drug or chemical is known, specific therapies need to be commenced (a summary of common drugs and antidotes can be found in Table 10.1). If the antidote is unknown then TOXBASE R or the National Poisons Information Service (NPIS) should be contacted for advice. Resuscitation may be required for several hours.

Thrombosis (pulmonary embolism or coronary thrombosis)

There may be a history of recent surgery, prolonged immobility or long-haul air travel. Vigorous chest compressions may be of use in breaking up a pulmonary embolism (PE). Thrombolytic therapy (Ruiz-Bailen et al. 2001, Caldicott et al. 2002, ILCOR 2005) should be considered if a PE is suspected, and resuscitation efforts continued for up to 90 min after administration. Urgent embolectomy is rarely used outside the setting of a cardiothoracic surgical centre.

CEASING A RESUSCITATION ATTEMPT

The decision to cease resuscitation events in hospital is usually made by the resuscitation team leader, taking into account the views of colleagues involved in the patient's care. In the community, paramedics and technicians are able to identify patients in whom resuscitation would be futile and distressing and survival is unlikely, using guidelines published by the Joint Royal Colleges Ambulance Liaison Committee (JRCALC 2004).

The duration of a resuscitation attempt will vary and be dependent on many factors, e.g. the interval between onset of cardiac arrest and start of BLS, the delay in ALS provision, and the patient's past history including any terminal illness. Decisions about ceasing a resuscitation attempt should not be made on the basis of the patient's age alone. Sedation preceding a cardiac arrest may protect against the effects of hypoxia, suggesting a need for prolonged resuscitation (Colquhoun et al. 2004). Hypothermia may also affect the length of time spent attempting resuscitation: death should not be confirmed until attempts are made to warm the patient as hypothermia can mimic death (Resuscitation Council (UK) 2002). Resuscitation in such 'special circumstances' is, however, outside the scope of this chapter and the reader is encouraged to seek detailed advice from appropriate sources.

POST-RESUSCITATION CARE

The return of spontaneous circulation and/or respiratory effort does not signal the end of the event. The resuscitation team cannot simply 'walk away' and leave others to provide ongoing care. The immediate post-resuscitation phase may be crucial to determining the outlook for the patient. Immediate assessments of vital functions need to be made: the ABC (airway, breathing, circulation) of resuscitation requires ongoing assessment:

- Is the patient able to maintain his or her own airway and breathe spontaneously?
- Are the heart rate and rhythm normal?
- What does the 12-lead ECG show?
- Is blood pressure stable?
- Is the patient warm and well perfused?
- Is the patient in pain or otherwise distressed?
- Are immediate interventions such as coronary angiography or thrombolysis indicated?

Assessment of ABC should be followed rapidly by assessment of D (disability) and E (exposure). For D, conscious level is assessed immediately using the AVPU system (American College of Surgeons 1997) or Glasgow Coma Scale (Teasdale and Jennett 1974). Exposure entails a full physical examination of the patient to ensure that nothing of significance (e.g. trauma or bleeding causing, or resulting from, the arrest or resuscitation attempt) has been missed. Blood samples should be sent for assessment of biochemistry (e.g. urea and electrolytes), arterial blood gases used to evaluate adequacy of ventilation and so forth, and biomarkers of myocardial damage such as troponins measured as judged appropriate by the senior clinician. A chest radiograph will also be necessary, especially if CPR has been performed and central lines or drains inserted. A urinary catheter and other interventions may be required to facilitate subsequent monitoring. It is important to communicate with the patient, to reassure him or her in what will inevitably be a time of great stress and anxiety. Loved ones will also require sensitive support and information.

Recent research has suggested that mild hypothermia maintained for 12–24 h after a cardiac arrest may improve outcome (Bernard et al. 2002). Consequently, it is recommended that unconscious adult patients who have regained spontaneous circulation after an out-of-hospital VF arrest should be cooled to 32–34°C (Nolan et al. 2003) and that some patients with other ECG rhythms surviving out-of-hospital cardiac arrest may also benefit. Abella et al. (2005) suggest that hypothermia is underused in post-resuscitation care.

THE ETHICS OF RESUSCITATION: END-OF-LIFE DECISIONS AND 'DO NOT ATTEMPT RESUSCITATION'

A successful resuscitation attempt is a wonderful outcome for most patients in whom it occurs, their loved ones, and those who have been involved in providing care. But a balance needs to be struck between this success, which is the exception rather than the rule (the majority of resuscitation attempts fail), and exposure of patients to the indignity of a vigorous resuscitation attempt when the likelihood of success is very low, or futile. The worst-case scenario might be a patient who survives with spontaneous breathing and circulation, but in a persistent vegetative state. The issues involved are complex and emotive and are discussed in detail by Baskett et al. (2005) and in guidance published by the British Medical Association, Resuscitation Council (UK) and Royal College of Nursing (2002).

Cultural, religious, ethical, societal, legal, familial, economic, scientific and other factors all arguably play a part in decisions about resuscitation. The time window for decision-making is often measured in seconds, particularly in the community where the role of 'do not attempt resuscitation' (DNAR) orders and living wills are only recently emerging, compared with the more formal setting of the hospital ward or the long-term care home. Health professionals are required to balance the benefits and risks of their actions, while trying always to do no harm. The wishes of the mentally competent patient (there should be a presumption of competence until demonstrated otherwise) must be respected. Patients and relatives do not have the right automatically to demand resuscitation when, for example, the responsible clinician judges such an attempt futile. Decisions, which should ideally be made by the most senior doctor involved in the patient's care, should be formally documented and regularly reviewed in light of changes in the patient's condition and expressed wishes. The views of family members, loved ones and members of the team providing care should be taken into consideration but, at present, are not binding on the ultimate (medical) decision-maker. In the absence of information to the contrary, the presumption is in favour of a resuscitation attempt (British Medical Association, Resuscitation Council (UK) and Royal College of Nursing 2002).

CONCLUSION

Despite four decades and more of experience with providing CPR, most patients who suffer a cardiac arrest do not survive. Recent changes to guidelines based on an international consensus of the available scientific evidence have attempted to simplify the process of resuscitation and highlighted the importance of continuing chest compressions with minimal 'time off chest'; 'compression-only' CPR, at least in the initial phase, is considered acceptable. Safety of the rescuer is paramount and there is growing appreciation that preventing cardiac arrest may be possible if certain warning signs result in appropriate corrective action. The ethical and legal background in which resuscitation decisions are made continues to evolve. The reader is encouraged to undertake formal (refresher) training in CPR on at least an annual basis, and to look to their local resuscitation training officer, the Resuscitation Council (UK) guidelines and related sources for detailed information on this fascinating area of practice.

REFERENCES

Abella B, Rhee J, Huang K et al. (2005) Induced hypothermia is underused after resuscitation from cardiac arrest: a current practice survey. *Resuscitation* **64**: 181–6.

American College of Surgeons (1997) *Student Course Manual.* Chicago: American College of Surgeons' Committee on Trauma.

Bahr J, Kingler H, Panzer W et al. (1997) Skills of lay people in checking the carotid pulse. *Resuscitation* **35**(1): 23–6.

Baskett PJ, Steen PA, Bossaert L (2005) European Resuscitation Council guidelines for resuscitation 2005. Section 8. The ethics of resuscitation and end-of-life decisions. *Resuscitation* **67**(suppl 1): S171–80.

Berg R, Hilwig R, Kern K, Ewy G (2000) Bystander chest compressions and assisted ventilation independently improve outcome from piglet asphyxia pulseless cardiac arrest. *Circulation* **101**: 1743–8.

Bernard S, Buist M, Safar P, Kockanek P (2002) Mild Therapeutic hypothermia to improve the neurologic outcome after cardiac arrest. *New England Journal of Medicine* **346**: 549–56.

British Medical Association, Resuscitation Council (UK) and Royal College of Nursing (2002) *Decisions Relating to Cardiopulmonary Resuscitation: A joint statement from the British Medical Association, Resuscitation Council (UK) and Royal College of Nursing.* London: BMA, Resuscitation Council (UK) and RCN.

Buist M, Moore G, Bernard S et al. (2002) Effects of emergency team on reduction of incidence of and mortality from unexpected cardiac arrests in hospital: Preliminary study. *British Medical Journal* **324**: 387–90.

Caldicott D, Parasivam S, Harding J et al. (2002) Tenecteplase for massive pulmonary embolism. *Resuscitation* **55**: 211–13.

Chellel A (2000) *Resuscitation. A guide for nurses.* London: Churchill Livingstone.

Colquhoun M, Handley A, Evans T (2004) *ABC of Resuscitation*, 5th edn. London: BMJ Books.

Cummins R, Ornato J, Thies W, Pepe P (1991) Improving survival from sudden cardiac arrest: the 'chain of survival' concept. A statement for health professionals from the Advanced Cardiac Life Support Subcommittee and the Emergency Cardiac Care Committee, American Heart Association. *Circulation* **83**: 1832–47

Davies CS, Colquhoun MC, Boyle R, Chamberlain DA (2005) A national programme for on-site defibrillation by lay people in selected high risk areas: initial results. *Heart* **91**: 1299–302

Engdahl J, Bang A, Lindquist J, Herlitz J (2001) Factors affecting short and long term prognosis among 1069 patients with out of hospital cardiac arrest and pulseless electrical activity. *Resuscitation* **51**: 17–25.

Gabbott D, Smith G, Mitchell S et al. (2005) Cardiopulmonary resuscitation standards for clinical practice and training in the UK. *Resuscitation* **64**: 13–19

Grayling M, Wilson I, Thomas B (2002) The use of the laryngeal mask airway and the combitube in cardiopulmonary resuscitation; a national survey. *Resuscitation* **55**: 171–5.

Gwinnutt CL, Columb M, Harris R (2000) Outcome after cardiac arrest in adults in UK hospitals: effect of the 1997 guidelines. *Resuscitation* **47**: 125–35.

Handley A (2002) Teaching hand placement for chest compression- a simpler technique. *Resuscitation* **53**: 29–36.

Handley A, Koster R, Monsieurs K et al. (2005) European resuscitation council guidelines for resuscitation 2005. Section 2. Adult basic life support and use of automated external defibrillators. *Resuscitation* **67**(suppl 1): S7–23.

International Liaison Committee on Resuscitation (ILCOR) (2005) Part 4 Advanced Life Support. *Resuscitation* **67**: 213–47.

Jevon P (2002) *Advanced Cardiac Life Support. A practical guide.* Oxford: Butterworth-Heinemann.

Joint Royal Colleges Ambulance Liaison Committee (2004) *Clinical Practice Guidelines.* Available from www.asancep.org.uk/JRCALC/guidelines/

Jowett N, Thompson D (2003) *Comprehensive Coronary Care*, 3rd edn. London: Elsevier Science.

Kerber R, Robertson C (1996) Transthoracic impedance. In: Paradis N, Halperin H, Nowark R (eds), *Cardiac Arrest: The science and practice of resuscitation medicine.* London. Williams & Wilkins, pp 481–94.

Kouwenhoven WB, Jude JR (1960) Closed chest massage. *Journal of American Medical Association* **173**: 1064–7.

Larsen M, Eisenberg M, Cummins R, Hallstrom A (1993) Predicting survival from out of hospital cardiac arrest: a graphic model. *Annals of Emergency Medicine* **22**: 1652–8.

Moule P, Albarran J (2005) *Practical Resuscitation: Recognition and response. (Essential Skills for Nursing).* Oxford: Blackwell Publishing.

Nolan J (1998) The 1998 European Resuscitation Guidelines for the adult single rescuer basic life support. *British Medical Journal* **316**: 1870–6.

Nolan J, Morley P, Vanden Hoek T, Hickey, and ALS Task Force (2003). Therapeutic hypothermia after cardiac arrest: An advisory statement by the Advanced Life Support Task Force of the International Liaison Committee on Resuscitation. *Resuscitation* **57**: 221–326.

Peberdy M, Kaye W, Ornato J et al. (2003) Cardiopulmonary resuscitation of adults in the hospital: A report of 14720 cardiac arrests from the national registry of cardiopulmonary resuscitation. *Resuscitation* **58**: 297–308.

Perkins G, Stephenson B, Hulme J, Monsieurs K (2005) Birmingham assessment of breathing study (BABS). *Resuscitation* **64**: 109–13.

Quinn T, Hatchett R (2002) Cardiopulmonary resuscitation in adults. In: Hatchett R, Thompson D (eds), *Cardiac Nursing: A comprehensive guide.* Edinburgh. Churchill Livingstone.

Resuscitation Council (UK) (2000) *Resuscitation Guidelines 2000.* London: Resuscitation Council (UK).

Resuscitation Council (UK) (2002) *Advanced Life Support Course Provider Manual*, 4th edn. London: Resuscitation Council (UK).

Resuscitation Council (UK) (2005) *Resuscitation Guidelines 2005.* London: Resuscitation Council (UK).

Resuscitation Council (UK) (2006) *Advanced Life Support*, 5th edn. London: Resuscitation Council (UK).

Ruiz-Bailen M, Aguayo de Hoyos, Serrano-Corcoles et al. (2001) Thrombolysis with recombinant tissue plasminogen activator during cardiopulmonary resuscitation in fulminant pulmonary embolism. *Resuscitation* **51**: 97–101.

Teasdale G, Jennett B (1974) Assessment of coma and impaired consciousness: a practical scale. *Lancet* **ii**: 81–4.

Waalewijn R, De Vos R, Tijssen J, Koster R (2001) Survival models for out of hospital cardiopulmonary resuscitation from the perspectives of the bystander, the first responder, and the paramedic. *Resuscitation* **51**: 113–22.

11 Congenital heart disease

LIZ SMITH

Congenital heart disease is a collective term for a range of malformations and defects that arise during embryonic and fetal development of the heart. The malformations and defects can be simple or complex and can occur in isolation or associated with abnormalities of other systems. Diagnosis and treatment of congenital heart disease have progressed and improved rapidly over the last few decades and therefore many affected infants are now surviving into adulthood. This has, in turn, led to a need for the development of services and expertise in the care of older children, adolescents and adults with congenital heart disease, many of whom have experienced complex surgical interventions for their abnormality. This chapter aims to explore the possible processes of congenital disease, the more common abnormalities, and the physiological, psychological and social needs of adolescents and adults who survive the effects and treatment of congenital heart disease. Surgical interventions for specific abnormalities will not be considered, because this is a very specialist field that is often tailored to the unique and specific needs of each patient's defect.

THE DEVELOPMENT OF THE HEART

The development of the heart begins very early in embryonic life. After fertilisation takes place there is rapid cell division to form a blastocyst, which then organises the inner cells into a group of cells known as the embryoblast whereas the outer cells become the trophoblast, which will later form the placenta. The embryoblast divides into three layers of cells: ectoderm, endoderm and mesoderm. Ectoderm will form the skin and nervous system; endoderm will form the inner lining of the gut, respiratory system and the glandular tissue of the liver and pancreas, etc.; and mesoderm will form the muscles and connective tissue of the head, trunk and skeletal system, and also gives rise to the cardiovascular system (Witt 1997). The heart forms from two endocardial tubes, which are brought together in the thoracic region by folding of the growing embryonic tissue. The two tubes fuse together and this fused area will

Cardiac Care: An Introduction for Healthcare Professionals. Edited by David Barrett, Mark Gretton and Tom Quinn
© 2006 John Wiley & Sons Ltd

form the heart itself whereas the non-fused tubes above and below will form the great vessels.

This creation of a primitive heart occurs around 20 days after conception. The heart is fixed in place and as the now single tube grows it folds on itself; this folding generally takes place from right to left, placing the heart in the left side of the chest. If folding for some reason takes place from left to right then the heart will be situated in the right side of the chest, i.e. dextrocardia (Matsumura and England 1992). Once folding is complete, around 28 days after conception, the heart begins to divide into chambers that are complete by around the end of the seventh week. Following this the major vessels develop to link with the appropriate chamber and valve leaflets form. The conduction system of the heart becomes functional by about 10 weeks and by 16 weeks sinus rhythm can be seen.

FETAL CIRCULATION

As the growing baby is reliant on the placenta for nutrition and gaseous exchange the circulation *in utero* has to be different to allow for this. Oxygenated blood enters the circulation from the placenta via the umbilical veins and thus into the inferior vena cava. This has the effect that oxygen saturation *in utero* is never higher than 65% so the fetus has a high red cell count to ensure maximum oxygen-carrying capacity. It also causes oxygenated blood to enter the right side of the heart rather than the left, as in extrauterine circulation. To accommodate this, the heart has two structures that allow right-to-left shunting: the foramen ovale between the atria and the ductus arteriosus between the aorta and the pulmonary artery. Right-to-left shunting is facilitated by the fact that the lungs are collapsed and therefore the vessels are coiled and tortuous, causing high vascular resistance. There is little circulation to the lungs because blood follows the path of least resistance across the foramen ovale and the ductus arteriosus. There is, however, sufficient circulation to oxygenate and nourish the lung tissue that continues growing and developing throughout intrauterine life (Witt 1997).

ADAPTATION TO EXTRAUTERINE LIFE

The transition from fetal circulation to extrauterine circulation takes about 7–10 days after birth. The lungs expand with the first breaths and there is an associated fall in pulmonary vascular resistance. The umbilical cord is cut and systemic blood pressure rises. The increased flow of blood to the lungs and back to the left atrium results in a change of pressure within the heart, which causes the 'trapdoor' of the foramen ovale to close; this occurs within 24–48 hours of birth. Changes in flow and pressure also cause minimal flow in the ductus arteriosus. The oxygen saturations rise to normal limits as the extrauterine circulation takes over, causing a fall in the production of prostaglandin E_2 which results in closure of the ductus during the first 7–10 days of life. The ductus is usually obliterated by 3 weeks of age.

CAUSES OF CONGENITAL HEART DISEASE

In common with many congenital defects the cause is obscure; however, there are some known predisposing factors. The most commonly known factor is maternal viral infection, particularly rubella (German measles). As the heart develops so early in intrauterine life, it is particularly vulnerable to damage from viruses that can be contracted before the woman even realises that she is pregnant and needs to take extra precautions to avoid infection. The incidence of rubella-related abnormalities has, however, been reduced by routine immunisation of adolescent girls. Another major factor in the incidence of congenital heart disease in the modern world is alcohol. Up to 30% of infants with fetal alcohol syndrome will have an associated heart defect. It was thought that the syndrome occurred only when the mother drank excessively and regularly, as in alcoholism. However, the increased incidence of fetal alcohol syndrome in the USA has prompted further research into the amounts of alcohol associated with damage to the fetus. Meanwhile the advice to pregnant women continues to be abstinence. This advice may not be effective in reducing the incidence of heart defects because of the early development of the cardiovascular system and the culture of binge drinking in young women.

It is thought that the taking of some drugs may predispose to congenital heart disease. There are careful controls in place for the prescription of drugs in pregnancy to avoid harm from teratogenic medicines, but it is not always possible to ensure the absolute safety of drugs, as thalidomide has shown. Generally, women who take regular prescriptions are advised to seek preconceptual advice about their therapy. The rising use of recreational drugs has not yet been adequately researched in relation to congenital abnormalities, but this is clearly an area for concern, particularly in the UK where teenage pregnancy rates are high.

Maternal age has also been shown to have an influence on the incidence of congenital heart disease. Pregnancies at either end of the reproductive age range are more at risk. This is an area of concern given the modern trend for women to start their families much later than in previous generations, but is also a concern given the high teenage pregnancy rates, particularly in areas of social deprivation. Maternal disease, notably diabetes, has been associated with an increased risk of congenital heart disease. However, better management of chronic disease and glycaemic control in diabetes have reduced the risk significantly. There is also a strong link between chromosomal disorders of the infant and congenital heart disease. About 40% of babies with Down syndrome will have an associated heart defect. This has in the past raised much ethical debate about treatment for these infants, but it is now generally accepted that they have the right to the same interventions as chromosomally normal children. There is now recognition of genetic causes of congenital heart disease. Congenital heart defects have been an acknowledged part of some genetic syndromes; however, it is becoming apparent that some non-syndromic defects have a genetic cause (Hinton et al. 2005).

COMMON CONGENITAL HEART DEFECTS

The presentation of congenital heart disease is complex and it is impossible to address all the types and combinations of defects here. The more common defects are therefore described to provide a flavour of the problems and clinical findings in affected children.

ATRIAL SEPTAL DEFECT

Atrial septal defects (ASDs) are gaps in the septum between the two atria, which are commonly associated with an anomaly in development of the area of tissue that forms the foramen ovale *in utero*. This defect is twice as common in girls as it is in boys and occurs in about 1 in 1500 live births. ASDs often go undiagnosed until adulthood when medical checks may detect a murmur. There is an associated risk of atrial dysrhythmia in later life in unrepaired defects, and adult repairs are now being undertaken. Infants who have the defect diagnosed generally tolerate it well and will undergo surgical repair between 2 and 4 years of age. Repair will be by direct suture or patch as required. As many adults with an ASD may be asymptomatic it is important to consider the possible presence of this anomaly when evaluating patients for unrelated cardiac interventions, particularly transvenous pacing, because there is an increased risk of strokes and other embolic events (Webb 2003).

VENTRICULAR SEPTAL DEFECT

These defects vary in size from a pinhole to complete absence of a septum; however, many of the smaller anomalies are thought to close spontaneously in the first year of life. Pressure in the left ventricle will cause left-to-right shunting in the larger defects and this will lead to higher pulmonary vascular resistance and right ventricular hypertrophy, and then ultimately cardiac failure. Surgical closure will therefore be necessary for larger defects, generally between 2 and 4 years of age; however, if the child is failing to thrive closure will be performed earlier. Ventricular septal defects (VSDs) occur in between 1.5 and 3.5 per 1000 live births and affect both males and females equally. It is a disorder that is frequently associated with other defects.

TRANSPOSITION OF THE GREAT VESSELS

Transposition involves the major arteries arising from the wrong ventricle, i.e. the aorta originates in the right ventricle and the pulmonary artery from the left side. The result of this is two closed circulatory systems except for the connection across the ductus arteriosus. Indeed it is the ductus that sustains circulation unless a VSD is also present. The defect is therefore termed 'duct dependent' and initial treatment is with an infusion of prostaglandin E to maintain the patency of the ductus. This is the most commonly diagnosed heart defect in the newborn period. The affected infant will present with cyanosis either on feeding or on crying because oxygenation is inadequate for activity. Initial treatment is palliative, generally by the creation of a VSD by balloon septostomy. Surgery to correct the defect involves either atrial switch (Mustard or Senning procedures) or more recently, arterial switch.

TETRALOGY OF FALLOT

This is a collection of four defects: VSD, pulmonary artery valve stenosis, overriding aorta (i.e. the aorta arises from a central point and receives blood from both ventricles) and right ventricular hypertrophy. The VSD is usually large, so the haemodynamics of this disorder depend on the degree of pulmonary valve stenosis and the pulmonary and systemic vascular resistance. Tetralogy is the most common cyanotic defect and accounts for 10–15% of all cases of congenital heart disease. Some infants may be severely cyanosed at birth, but more commonly, affected children suffer increasing cyanosis in the first year of life as pulmonary valve stenosis worsens. Anoxic episodes will occur when the child's oxygen requirements increase, e.g. when crying or feeding. Repair of this defect requires closure of the VSD and dilatation or incision of the pulmonary valve to improve right ventricular outflow.

COARCTATION OF THE AORTA

This involves localised narrowing of the aortic arch near the insertion of the ductus arteriosus. It causes increased pressure before the narrowing and lower pressure beyond it; this results in a higher blood pressure in the arms, often with an associated bounding pulse, a lower blood pressure in the legs, and a weak or absent femoral pulse. Infants who present with coarctation will do so shortly after closure of the ductus arteriosus. They will demonstrate inadequate systemic perfusion, severe acidosis and hypoglycaemia, and therefore require urgent resuscitation. Older children and adults may be diagnosed because of weak femoral pulses. Checking femoral pulses has become an important element in the examination of the newborn. Severe coarctation will need surgery in early infancy, otherwise it will be undertaken when the child is older (often between 3 and 10 years of age). This defect has commonly been thought of as an isolated, simple anomaly but is now thought of as part of a diffuse arteriopathy with a tendency to aneurysm (Warnes 2005). Ascending aortic aneurysm is a commonly encountered complication of the condition and systemic hypertension despite repair has been found to occur in up to 75% of patients (Warnes 2005).

HYPOPLASTIC LEFT HEART SYNDROME

This condition is characterised by hypoplasia of the left ventricle in association with atresia or stenosis of the aortic valve, atresia or stenosis of the mitral valve and hypoplasia of the aortic arch. The syndrome accounts for only about 1% of congenital defects; however, it is responsible for 25% of the cardiac deaths in the first week of life. The condition is 'duct dependent' because systemic circulation is reliant on right-to-left shunting across the ductus. Severe tachypnoea and cyanosis develop within the first 72 hours of life. Without treatment the condition is fatal although treatment itself is not without some controversy. Surgical repair is complex and in three stages. Surgery is a relatively recent intervention and was developed in the USA, and it is not clear how long surviving children will be able to live without a heart transplantation; indeed should surgery fail then transplantation is the only option. The change from conservative medical management of the condition to aggressive surgical interventions has caused ethical debate, particularly as donor hearts are not always available and success cannot be guaranteed. However, as the condition would otherwise be fatal many parents choose to risk surgery.

ADOLESCENTS AND ADULTS WITH CONGENITAL HEART DISEASE

The improvements made in recognising and treating congenital heart disease have resulted in many more affected patients surviving into adulthood. These patients can present as cardiac or non-cardiac patients within the healthcare system, and they need specialised care to manage their individual needs. Treating congenital heart disease does not always result in 'normal' or even near-normal cardiac function, and surgical interventions will have effects over and above the direct repair of the defect. In addition to this, patients with congenital heart disease have unique psychosocial needs. These patients do not always easily 'fit' into existing cardiology services because their needs are so very different from those of most cardiac patients. As a result, adolescents often remain with paediatric services far longer than is perhaps appropriate, and the transition to adult care is not always easy for them. However, specialist services are now being developed to address this problem. The next section discusses the complications of congenital heart disease in adolescents and adults and their subsequent care needs wherever they may be cared for within the healthcare services.

ARRHYTHMIAS

Arrhythmias are a cause of mortality and morbidity in adolescent and adult congenital heart disease patients, possibly even causing sudden death. Patients should be educated to report any palpitations, dizziness or syncope promptly because hospital admission for assessment is necessary (Alderman 2000, British Cardiac Society 2002). For detailed discussion of the arrhythmias below, see Chapter 9. Treatment of arrhythmia in this group of patients requires specialist knowledge to prevent complications and also because of the difficulties of treating patients with non-standard cardiac anatomy (British Cardiac Society 2002).

Sinus node disease may occur as a result of surgery involving the atrium (e.g. transposition) and, although this is often identified in the early post-operative period, it can take months or years for dysfunction to occur. Atrioventricular block occurs in up to 75% of patients with corrected transposition, but also can occur in patients who have experienced surgery to the ventricular septum (Silka and McAnulty 1997).

Atrial arrhythmias, particularly atrial flutter, are an important cause of mortality and morbidity in adult congenital heart disease patients. Patients will present with dizziness or syncope, palpitations, chest pain on effort or hepatic discomfort. The problem is part of the natural history of certain defects or may be the result of surgical scarring (British Cardiac Society 2002). Atrial fibrillation may occur in patients with a previously asymptomatic ASD in later life. Re-entry tachycardias may occur in some patients, particularly those with a corrected transposition (Silka and McAnulty 1997). Ventricular arrhythmias may occur as a result of either the natural history of the defect or the surgical interventions, and may not appear until years after surgery.

INFECTIVE ENDOCARDITIS

Most patients with congenital heart disease have a life-long risk of endocarditis, which has a mortality rate of about 20% (Alderman 2000, British Cardiac Society 2002). As a result of the high mortality and morbidity, it is important that the disease be detected promptly; delay in diagnosis and referral is common and is often because physical signs may be difficult to interpret. Dental hygiene is vital to reduce the risk, so regular dental care must be strongly recommended and encouraged. It is also important that patients are educated about the serious risks associated with tattoos, body piercing and acupuncture. Tattoos and body piercing are particularly popular with younger people, who may experience peer pressure, so sensitive health education is essential. From a healthcare perspective, however, it is also important that staff caring for these patients in non-cardiac situations understand the risks associated with invasive monitoring, intravenous cannulation and urinary catheters. Prophylactic antibiotic therapy will be necessary for most patients who require such interventions; however, it must be recognised that this does not always prevent endocarditis (British Cardiac Society 2002).

RISKS ASSOCIATED WITH PROSTHETIC MATERIALS

Risks will vary according to the nature and type of the prosthetic material; however, thromboembolism and endocarditis are associated with prosthetic valves. As a result of the thromboembolic risk, these patients are often on anticoagulants, which makes bleeding a problem so health education in this respect is vital. Prosthetics will need replacing and the major surgery involved clearly holds risks for these patients. The life of a prosthetic valve depends on whether it was inserted in childhood (when it may need replacing because it is no longer big enough) and the material used (Alderman 2000).

RISKS ASSOCIATED WITH CYANOTIC DEFECTS

Reduced glomerular filtration rate, proteinuria and hyperuricaemia may occur because of long-standing hypoxaemia, culminating in renal impairment. There may also be associated gouty arthritis. Fluid balance is essential because patients are at risk of renal insufficiency and heart failure, particularly after surgery. Patients are also at more significant risk of sepsis (Alderman 2000).

Patients with cyanotic defects are at a greater risk than non-cyanotic patients of cerebrovascular embolic events, particularly in the presence of hypertension or atrial fibrillation. Anti-embolic care is essential postoperatively and health education in relation to not standing or sitting for long periods and crossing the legs is an important element of care. Central lines should be avoided where possible and filters should always be used with intravenous lines (Webb 2003).

Erythrocytosis can occur as a compensation mechanism for the decreased oxygen saturation caused by the cyanotic defect. The increase in red blood cells causes an increase in viscosity and associated problems. These patients have a higher risk of gallstones and acute cholecystitis because of the higher than normal red cell count. Other symptoms that may be experienced include dizziness, headaches, fatigue, muscle aches and weakness, and tinnitus (Alderman 2000). Health education in relation to avoiding dehydration, which will exacerbate hyperviscosity and nutrition, is important for these patients (Webb 2003).

Eisenmenger's syndrome is a progressive and potentially fatal pulmonary vascular disease found in patients with intracardiac shunting (Alderman 2000). Patients with this diagnosis may die at any time and should be monitored to anticipate and prevent health threats. Any surgical intervention or anaesthetic must be planned carefully (Webb 2003).

PSYCHOSOCIAL CARE NEEDS

Successful treatment of congenital heart disease cannot simply be about prolonging life but also about improving the quality of life (Lane et al. 2002). There has therefore got to be a strong psychosocial element within the care of these patients to ensure that they get the most out of their lives, despite inevitable restrictions. Recent research suggests that psychosocial needs of congenital heart disease patients are not being met and that this adversely affects normal adolescent/adult development and relationships (Lyon et al 2005). Each individual patient will have his or her own unique needs and more research is required into this aspect of care, but issues requiring support can include body image, sexuality and reproduction, and lifestyle changes.

Increasingly in western society there is an emphasis on appearance, particularly in young people and for females. Corrective surgery for congenital heart disease can leave the patients with significant scarring and this may have a negative effect on the patient's body image, to the extent that it affects their ability to establish relationships and to socialise generally. Cyanotic patients may be all too aware of the effect that this has on their overall appearance. In addition to the physical body image, patients may also be affected by their inability to participate in the activities of their peers; this is particularly difficult for adolescents who may want to be involved in sports, dancing and other leisure pursuits. Expert counselling and support must therefore be provided to help patients deal with these feelings and to find activities that are possible for them (British Cardiac Society 2002). Practical advice with respect to what is possible in terms of physical and sporting activity is essential because patients often have limited understanding of the implications of their condition and may try to do either more or less than is possible. This is a particularly relevant area that requires further research given the recent evidence that links exercise capacity with well-being (Lane et al. 2002).

Expert advice is essential in respect to contraception because this is a particularly difficult area for the woman with congenital heart disease. More open dialogue about sexuality and contraception needs to start in adolescence and continue throughout adulthood (Miner 2004). Oral contraception may well be contraindicated for many patients; however, the mini-pill may be appropriate for some women (Cannobbio et al. 2005). Sterilisation may be problematic because of the risks of anaesthesia and surgery. Congenital heart disease is now the most common cardiac-related cause of mortality and morbidity in pregnancy and childbirth. It is essential that all women be provided with genetic counselling, and advice with respect to complications and the fetal risk from maternal complications. Care should be closely coordinated between the cardiologist and obstetrician (British Cardiac Society 2002). There are now more data available to advise women about the risks of pregnancy, but this remains a complex area of care (Cannobbio 2004). Generally, clinically stable patients tolerate pregnancy well. Genetic advice is also important for male patients.

Patients with congenital heart disease will need sensitive health education to ensure that they enjoy as healthy a life as possible. Avoidance of cigarette smoking, excessive alcohol intake and use of recreational drugs is important. Nutritional advice to avoid obesity and complications related to their condition is vital. Specific advice may also be necessary in respect of sexual activity, complementary therapies, and body piercing and tattoos. Insurance and mortgages can be difficult or even impossible to obtain for this group of patients. Support from specialists can be valuable in this respect. It should also be noted that support and advice can be obtained from the Grown Up Congenital Heart (GUCH) Patients' Association.

CONCLUSION

Patients who survive congenital heart disease are a growing population as diagnosis and treatment techniques develop and improve. Accurate figures are not available but about 80–85% of patients will survive to adulthood (16 years) (British Cardiac Society 2002). Services for these patients are not yet well developed and recommendations for care provision have been made by the British Cardiac Society Working Party, chaired by Professor Jane Somerville. It is essential that the specialist needs of these patients are recognised and that their health and well-being are not compromised by substandard care. These patients will have care needs unrelated to the cardiac disease and it is therefore important that all healthcare professionals seek advice from specialists with regard to effective care management.

REFERENCES

Alderman L (2000) At risk: Adolescents and adults with congenital heart disease. *Dimensions of Critical Care Nursing* **19**(1): 2–12.

British Cardiac Society (2002) Grown-up congenital heart (GUCH) disease: current needs and provision of service for adolescents and adults with congenital heart disease in the UK. *Heart* **88** i1–14.

Cannobbio M (2004) Pregnancy in congenital heart disease: maternal risk. *Progress in Pediatric Cardiology* **19**(1): 1–3.

Cannobbio M, Perloff J, Rapkin A (2005) Gynecological health of females with congenital heart disease. *International Journal of Cardiology* **98**: 379–87.

Hinton R, Yutzey K, Woodrow, Benson D (2005) Congenital heart disease: Genetic causes and developmental insights. *Progress in Pediatric Cardiology* **20**: 101–11.

Lane D, Lip G, Millane T (2002) Quality of life in adults with congenital heart disease. *Heart* **88**: 71–5.
Lyon M, McCarter R, Kuehl K (2005) Transition to adulthood in congenital heart disease: Missed adolescent milestones. *Journal of Adolescent Health* **36**: 128.
Matsumura G, England M (1992) *Embryology Colouring Book*. London: Wolfe Publishing.
Miner PD (2004) Contraceptive choices for females with congenital heart disease. *Progress in Pediatric Cardiology* **19**: 15–24.
Silka M, McAnulty J (1997) Arrhythmias in patients with congenital heart disease. *Cardiac Electrophysiology Review* **1**(2): 237–40.
Warnes C (2005) The adult with congenital heart disease: Born to be bad? *Journal of the American College of Cardiology* **46**(1): 1–8.
Webb G (2003) Challenges in the care of adult patients with congenital heart defects. *Heart* 89: 465–9.
Witt C (1997) Cardiac embryology. *Neonatal Network* **16**(1): 43–9.

FURTHER READING

Brennan P, Young I (2001) Congenital heart malformations: aetiology and associations. *Seminars in Neonatology* **6**: 17–25.
Hay W, Hayward A, Levin M, Sondheimer J (eds) (1999) *Current Paediatric Diagnosis and Treatment*. Stamford, CA: Appleton & Lange.
Macnab A, Macrae D, Henning R (eds) (1999) *Care of the Critically Ill Child*. London: Churchill Livingstone.
Manning N, Archer N (2001) Treatment and outcome of serious structural congenital heart disease. *Seminars in Neonatology* **6**: 37–47.
Shinebourne E, Gatzoulis M (2002) Adult congenital heart disease. *Current Paediatrics* **12**: 220–6.

12 Valve disease, cardiomyopathy and inflammatory disorders

DAVID BARRETT

VALVE DISEASE

Valve disease usually falls into one of two categories: stenosis or regurgitation. All four of the valves in the heart can become diseased and cause morbidity and mortality. However, it is in the two valves on the left side of the heart – the mitral and aortic – that disease is most common and clinically significant.

MITRAL STENOSIS

Stenosis of the mitral valve occurs when the points at which the valve leaflets meet, known as the commissures, become diseased. The commissures fuse together as they become thickened and calcified over a period of years (Rahimtoola and Dell'Italia 2004). This disease process is almost always the result of the patient having had acute rheumatic fever earlier in life, causing recurrent inflammation of the valve. The decrease in rheumatic fever prevalence throughout the developed world has led to a gradual reduction in rates of mitral stenosis.

As the fusing of the valve leaflets progresses, the opening through which blood passes from the left atrium to the left ventricle diminishes in size. The narrower the valve opening becomes, the more difficult the expulsion of blood from the left atrium becomes. This results in the pressure within the left atrium rising and the walls of the atrium becoming stretched. The increase in left atrial pressure begins to back up, causing hypertension in the pulmonary circulation and compensatory enlargement of the right side of the heart (Yachimski and Lilly 2003).

Cardiac Care: An Introduction for Healthcare Professionals. Edited by David Barrett, Mark Gretton and Tom Quinn
© 2006 John Wiley & Sons Ltd

Signs, symptoms and diagnosis

Because mitral stenosis develops over a period of years, the onset of symptoms is usually rather gradual. Shortness of breath is a common manifestation of the disease, often caused by pulmonary oedema secondary to raised pressure in the pulmonary circulation. The enlarged left atrium can produce arrhythmias, causing palpitations and dizziness. Patients may also experience general symptoms such as tiredness and a productive cough (Rahimtoola and Dell'Italia 2004).

The medical history can provide a significant clue to the cause of symptoms. Any patient who has a history of rheumatic fever should be considered at high risk of mitral stenosis. However, it should be recognised that many patients may not know that they had rheumatic fever, so a failure to report this should not rule it out.

A number of investigations should be carried out to aid diagnosis. An electrocardiogram (ECG) will often show a characteristic notched P wave (sometimes called P mitrale). The chest radiograph is helpful in detecting any pulmonary oedema, and may also show enlargement of the left atrium. Echocardiography can show the structure and movement of the mitral valve, the size of the chambers of the heart and the rate at which blood passes through the narrowed opening. If echocardiography does not provide enough information about the disease, cardiac catheterisation can be performed to give accurate measurements of pressure differences between the left atrium and left ventricle (Blackburn and Bookless 2002).

Clinical management

Medical management of mitral stenosis focuses on supportive measures and prevention of complications. Pulmonary oedema can be resolved through the use of diuretics, and antibiotics are indicated if the patient has recurrent rheumatic fever (Rahimtoola and Dell'Italia 2004). The risks of arrhythmias secondary to left atrial enlargement can be reduced through the use of antiarrhythmic medication. Where arrhythmias are a risk, embolisation should also be considered as a potential problem, and oral anticoagulation should be started (Blackburn and Bookless 2002).

The only curative therapies for mitral stenosis involve physically repairing or replacing the valve. The valve can be opened with a balloon inserted percutaneously – a procedure called balloon mitral valvuloplasty (see Chapter 14 for more details). Alternatively, if the patient is not suitable for a valvuloplasty, the valve can be either repaired surgically or replaced with a prosthetic valve (see Chapter 15).

AORTIC STENOSIS

As discussed above, stenosis of a valve involves the fusion of the leaflets as a result of calcification, causing a narrowed opening through which blood can pass. In the case of aortic stenosis, it is the passage of blood from the left ventricle into the aorta that is obstructed. Although aortic stenosis can result as a complication of rheumatic fever, it is often simply a result of degenerative changes linked to the natural ageing process. The occurrence of aortic stenosis in young people is usually related to a congenital defect, apparent in up to 2% of the population, in which the aortic valve has two rather than three leaflets (Yachimski and Lilly 2003).

As narrowing of the aortic valve worsens, the pressure that the left ventricle must generate to expel blood has to increase steadily. The increased workload of the left ventricle causes the chamber to increase in size (undergo hypertrophy). The expansion in size of the left ventricle causes four main problems: first, the additional muscle mass and workload can cause excessive myocardial oxygen demand, leading to symptoms of angina; second, the enlarged ventricle may not be able to respond to a need for additional cardiac output whenever patients exert themselves. This may result in poor cerebral perfusion during exercise, leading to dizziness or even loss of consciousness. Thirdly, hypertrophy of the left ventricle can cause arrhythmias, with symptoms ranging from palpitations and dizziness through to sudden death. Finally, the abnormally enlarged left ventricle may become dysfunctional, leading to heart failure (Yachimski and Lilly 2003).

Signs, symptoms and diagnosis

The clinical manifestations of aortic stenosis are usually linked to the resulting left ventricular hypertrophy (LVH). The occurrence and severity of these signs and symptoms – chest pain, dizziness on exertion and breathlessness – will depend on the progression of the disease. As with all valve disorders, an ECG, chest radiograph and echocardiogram should be obtained. The ECG may show some non-specific abnormalities related to LVH, whereas chest radiography, echocardiography and cardiac catheterisation may allow visual confirmation of an enlarged left ventricle. In addition, echocardiography and cardiac catheterisation will allow for visual assessment of the movement of the aortic valve, and can be used to assess pressure differences between the left ventricle and aorta, often known as the gradient (Blackburn and Bookless 2002).

Clinical management

The central question in deciding on a treatment strategy for a patient with aortic stenosis is whether or not symptoms are present (Carabello 2002). If the patient is asymptomatic, as is often the case in mild or moderate disease, there may be no need for a regular medication regimen (Rahimtoola 2004). However, patients with aortic stenosis are at risk of developing infective endocarditis and should receive antibiotic prophylaxis when having certain invasive procedures (see below). Some lifestyle modification may be necessary for younger patients with aortic stenosis. The risk of exercise-related syncope, coupled with the potential for fatal arrhythmias, requires patients to avoid excessive physical activity (Blackburn and Bookless 2002). Importantly, the asymptomatic patient should be assessed at least annually to detect any deterioration.

Once a patient becomes symptomatic, the long-term prognosis without treatment is poor (Carabello 2002). As with mitral stenosis, corrective treatment can be carried out using an interventional cardiology technique called balloon valvuloplasty (see Chapter 14). However, in the case of aortic stenosis, this approach is suited only to certain groups of patients, notably those of a young age or those who are not suitable for aortic valve surgery (Rahimtoola 2004). For most patients with aortic stenosis, surgery is the most appropriate option. Depending on the condition of the aortic valve, the surgeon can opt to either repair the valve or replace it with a mechanical or biological prosthesis (see Chapter 15).

MITRAL REGURGITATION

Healthy cardiac valves will only allow blood flow in one direction. In the case of the mitral valve, blood flow is unidirectional from the left atrium into the left ventricle. Mitral regurgitation (MR) is the flow of some blood back into the left atrium from the left ventricle during ventricular systole.

There are many different causes of MR. One of the most common reasons is mitral valve prolapse, a degenerative disorder in which the leaflets of the valve become weakened and move into the left atrium during ventricular systole (Rahimtoola and Dell'Italia 2004). MR may be secondary to another disease process, such as rheumatic fever, hypertrophic cardiomyopathy or infective endocarditis (see below). Another possible cause of MR is coronary heart disease. Ischaemia or infarction of the papillary muscles that help to support the mitral valve can result in a loss of function. In rare cases, myocardial infarction can cause rupture of a papillary muscle, resulting in acute and severe MR (Blackburn and Bookless 2002).

Regurgitation of blood back into the left atrium causes a number of progressive changes to the structure and function of the heart. The pressure within the left atrium rises as a result of the additional blood volume. In acute MR, this sudden increase in left atrial pressure will back up into the pulmonary circulation, causing breathlessness and possibly pulmonary oedema (Yachimski and Lilly 2003). If the MR is chronic, the left atrium will adapt to the increased pressure by dilating, allowing for a greater volume of blood to be contained within it (Yachimski and Lilly 2003). Although this does decrease the pressure within the left atrium, it also increases the patient's risk of developing atrial fibrillation (Blackburn and Bookless 2002). Another consequence of MR is a potential reduction in cardiac output because, rather than blood from the left ventricle being expelled purely into the aorta, some is lost back into the left atrium. To compensate for this, the left ventricle contracts with greater force, to ensure that cardiac output is maintained at normal levels. However, if the left ventricle is subject to this increased workload over a long period of time, as is the case in chronic MR, it can become enlarged and eventually dysfunctional (Yachimski and Lilly 2003).

Signs, symptoms and diagnosis

The signs and symptoms of MR are usually a result of the pathophysiological mechanisms described above, i.e. increasing pressure within the left atrium in acute MR, and enlargement of the left atrium and left ventricle in chronic MR. In acute MR, the patient will often present with sudden-onset pulmonary oedema, characterised by breathlessness that is worsened by lying flat (orthopnoea). Patients with chronic disease will have a period of symptom onset over many years. These symptoms may include general tiredness and weakness related to an increasingly enlarged and dysfunctional left ventricle (Yachimski and Lilly 2003). Breathlessness will become more apparent as left ventricular failure develops, and the patient may develop atrial fibrillation causing palpitations and dizziness.

A chest radiograph may detect pulmonary oedema in patients with acute MR, or show enlargement of the left atrium and left ventricle in patients with chronic MR. An ECG is necessary to detect any arrhythmias, and might also indicate the presence of left ventricular enlargement (Rahimtoola and Dell'Italia 2004). Echocardiography is an important diagnostic tool in MR, because it allows visualisation of the jet of blood passing out of the left ventricle, through the diseased mitral valve and back into the left atrium. This type of scan can also allow for evaluation of the size of the affected chambers of the heart and detect abnormal movement of the mitral valve (Rahimtoola and Dell'Italia 2004). If echocardiography does not provide sufficient data, cardiac catheterisation can be performed to allow further assessment of myocardial and valve function.

Clinical management

There are no medical therapies that actually cure mitral regurgitation, but it may be possible to prevent or treat complications with medication. Patients who develop atrial fibrillation will require anti-arrhythmic therapy and anticoagulation. Prophylactic antibiotics may be required to prevent infective endocarditis and/or recurrence of underlying rheumatic fever (Otto 2003). Should symptoms of pulmonary congestion or left ventricular dysfunction manifest, these will require treatment with diuretics, nitrates and angiotensin-converting enzyme (ACE) inhibitors. Once symptoms are apparent and the disease has progressed from mild to moderate or severe, the need for surgical intervention, in the form of valve repair or replacement, should be urgently considered.

AORTIC REGURGITATION

The fundamental pathophysiology associated with aortic regurgitation (AR) is the same as that outlined for MR above – the flow of blood the wrong way through a cardiac valve. However, in AR, the abnormal blood flow is from the aorta into the left ventricle during diastole (Yachimski and Lilly 2003). As with all valve disorders, AR can be a complication of rheumatic fever or infective endocarditis. However, it is also often caused by abnormalities of the section of the aorta in which the valve is situated (often called the aortic root). In particular, AR can result from disease processes that cause enlargement of the aortic root, such as aortic aneurysm or dissection (Blackburn and Bookless 2002).

If AR develops acutely, the blood returning to the left ventricle from the aorta results in increased pressure during diastole. This increase in pressure in the left ventricle backs up into the left atrium and then into the pulmonary circulation, resulting in pulmonary oedema (Yachimski and Lilly 2003). In chronic AR, the left ventricle adapts to the gradually rising volume of blood returning from the aorta by increasing in size. The enlarged ventricle can accommodate greater volumes of blood, resulting in no increased pressures throughout the left side of the heart and the pulmonary circulation. Although this adaptive mechanism may initially prevent the patients from developing symptoms, the AR will continue to worsen. Eventually, the abnormally enlarged left ventricle will become dysfunctional, and signs of left ventricular failure will become apparent.

Signs, symptoms and diagnosis

Patients with acute AR will often present with severe, sudden-onset pulmonary oedema, characterised by shortness of breath, worse at night and when lying down. Symptoms of chronic AR may also include shortness of breath, but will develop gradually.

A characteristic finding when assessing a patient with AR is a large difference between the systolic and diastolic blood pressures – known as the pulse pressure. This is because the initial force of systole remains strong, but the regurgitation of blood from the aorta causes a sudden drop off in diastolic pressure (Yachimski and Lilly 2003). A chest radiograph will show significant left ventricular enlargement in patients with chronic AR, although this will probably not be present in patients with acute-onset disease. However, acute AR will usually result in pulmonary oedema that may be visible on a chest radiograph. Standard cardiac investigations should also include an ECG, which may show changes related to left ventricular enlargement. Echocardiography will allow assessment of left ventricular size, calculation of the scale of regurgitation and the anatomy of the aortic root. Cardiac catheterisation may also be necessary to provide additional detail of the scale of the disease and the function of the left ventricle (Blackburn and Bookless 2002).

Clinical management

Asymptomatic patients may require no treatment, but will need regular evaluation with echocardiography to monitor the disease progression. As with all valve disorders, patients should also be educated about the need for prophylactic antibiotics when undergoing invasive procedures, to prevent the development of infective endocarditis (Yachimski and Lilly 2003). Patients who develop symptoms related to pulmonary congestion or left ventricular failure should be treated with diuretics and ACE inhibitors (Boon and Bloomfield 2002). If patients have become symptomatic, surgical repair of the valve or replacement with a prosthetic valve is the only option that will improve the patient's prognosis.

CARDIOMYOPATHY

Diseases of the heart muscle that affect cardiac function are collectively known as cardiomyopathies (Cruickshank 2004). Although there are many different types of cardiomyopathy, the most commonly observed are dilated cardiomyopathy (DCM), hypertrophic cardiomyopathy (HCM), restrictive cardiomyopathy (RCM) and arrhythmogenic right ventricular cardiomyopathy (ARVC). These four conditions share some characteristics, but there are also significant differences in presentation of the patient and treatment strategies.

DILATED CARDIOMYOPATHY

In patients with DCM the left ventricle (and sometimes the right) becomes dilated, resulting in impaired contraction. The underlying cause of DCM is not always apparent. In some patients, a genetic predisposition to the disease is the only identifiable factor. In others, the disease may be the result of an infection such as myocarditis (see below) or abuse of certain substances such as alcohol (Chen et al. 2003). The fundamental problem resulting from ventricular dilatation is an impaired ability to contract. Cardiac output will therefore decrease as the disease progresses, leading to increased pressure within the chambers of the heart and pulmonary congestion. Dilatation of the ventricles can also cause valve dysfunction or cardiac arrhythmias, further exacerbating the patient's condition.

Signs, symptoms and diagnosis

As DCM develops, the patient will increasingly display signs and symptoms of heart failure. Some of these will result from compensatory mechanisms designed to enhance perfusion of vital organs, e.g. peripheral vasoconstriction will result in cold and clammy skin, and a tachycardia may be present. Many other signs and symptoms will arise directly as a result of reduced cardiac output and pulmonary congestion. Patients may report a long history of fatigue, with increasing breathlessness and dizziness, particularly on exertion (Cruickshank 2004). The chest radiograph of a patient with DCM will invariably show an enlarged heart. An ECG may demonstrate some abnormalities, such as a resting tachycardia, but these are not specific to DCM. A definitive diagnosis can be made with echocardiography, which will provide assessment of the size and function of the enlarged ventricle(s) (Wood and Picard 2004).

Clinical management

Some elements of the treatment plan for a patient with DCM are pharmacological, and relate mainly to the treatment of ventricular dysfunction. As with most patients presenting with heart failure, diuretics should be considered for fluid overload, ACE inhibitors may ease the burden on the left ventricle, and digoxin or β blockers may assist in slowing the ventricular rate (O'Donoghue 2002). Arrhythmias require suppression, usually with medication, and patients may require anticoagulation to prevent the formation of thrombi. In cases of potentially fatal ventricular arrhythmias, the patient may benefit from the insertion of an implantable cardioverter defibrillator (see Chapter 14). In severe cases, the only option for improving long-term prognosis may be cardiac transplantation. This option relies on suitability of the patient, and availability of a donor heart, so rates of transplantation are relatively low. Another option, usually utilised as a short-term measure while a patient is awaiting transplantation, is the surgical implantation of mechanical circulatory support (see Chapter 15).

Education and support are also important elements of the patient's management. Light exercise should be encouraged, although this should cease if the patient develops symptoms such as breathlessness, dizziness or chest pain (O'Donoghue 2002). Given that there is sometimes a genetic element to DCM, many patients and their families will require genetic counselling regarding the risks of transmitting or inheriting the disease (Cruickshank 2004).

HYPERTROPHIC CARDIOMYOPATHY

HCM is a disease typically characterised by thickening of the left ventricular wall and the interventricular septum, not resulting from another disease process such as hypertension or aortic stenosis. The disease is caused by a genetic abnormality. This can either occur as a result of a spontaneous genetic mutation or be inherited from a parent who carries the abnormal gene (Chen et al. 2003).

The enlargement of the left ventricular and septal myocardium has a number of implications for the patient. From a mechanical point of view, the enlarged myocardium can cause an obstruction to the outflow of blood from the left ventricle and into the aorta. When HCM causes obstruction of ventricular outflow, it is sometimes referred to as hypertrophic obstructive cardiomyopathy (HOCM). HCM can also cause mitral valve dysfunction, further hindering the passage of blood out of the left ventricle (Nishimura et al. 2004).

Aside from causing outflow obstruction in some patients, HCM also results in diastolic dysfunction, with the thickened myocardium unable to relax properly (O'Donoghue 2002). The combination of diastolic dysfunction and ventricular outflow obstruction causes raised left ventricular pressures, which subsequently result in increased myocardial oxygen demand, and raised pressures in the left atrium and pulmonary venous system (Chen et al. 2003). Aside from mechanical problems, the abnormal and enlarged myocardial cells can cause fatal arrhythmias such as ventricular fibrillation (O'Donoghue 2002).

Signs, symptoms and diagnosis

Many patients with HCM remain asymptomatic for a long period of time, with diagnosis being made only as a result of routine cardiac investigations or specific screening tests (Nishimura et al. 2004). Sudden death from a ventricular arrhythmia is often the first manifestation of HCM. Sudden death from HCM is often associated with young adults during exercise, and is the most common cause of sudden death in people under the age of 30 (Cruickshank 2004). In symptomatic patients, the most commonly reported manifestations of HCM are shortness of breath (caused by high pulmonary circulation pressure), chest pain (resulting from increased myocardial oxygen demand), and dizziness (caused by arrhythmias) (Chen et al. 2003).

The diagnosis of HCM is made through a combination of history and investigation. A family history of HCM makes the disease more likely in a patient and, in many cases, members of an HCM sufferer's family are routinely screened (Wigle 2001). A definitive diagnosis can be made using echocardiography to visualise the enlargement of the myocardium. Echocardiography can also enable assessment of whether or not HCM has resulted in left ventricular outflow obstruction, and can gauge the severity of the obstruction (Nishimura et al. 2004). Distinguishing between obstructive HCM and non-obstructive HCM is an important part of the diagnostic process because treatment strategies may be different. An ECG and chest radiograph should also be carried out, and these will usually demonstrate some non-specific abnormalities (O'Donoghue 2002).

Clinical management

In terms of medical therapy, β blockers are often administered to patients with HCM because they reduce heart rate (increasing the filling time for the ventricles), and lessen the force with which the ventricles contract, thereby reducing myocardial oxygen demand (Maron et al. 2003). It is also thought that by reducing the contractility of the left ventricle, β blockers can help to relieve the outflow obstruction to some degree (O'Donoghue 2002). If patients are unable to tolerate β blockers, or if they are contraindicated because of a history of asthma, the calcium channel blocker verapamil can be used. It should be noted that, in patients with severe HOCM, verapamil may worsen the condition, so the drug should be either used cautiously (Nishimura et al. 2004) or avoided all together (McKenna and Behr 2002).

The anti-arrhythmic agent disopyramide, which also has a negative effect on the force of cardiac contraction, has been shown to give some benefit when added to a β blocker (McKenna and Behr 2002). It should be noted that drugs leading to a reduction in blood volume (e.g. diuretics) should be used very cautiously because they can result in the worsening of any existing outflow obstruction (Chen et al. 2003). Nitrates, ACE inhibitors and digoxin should also be avoided in patients with HOCM (Maron et al. 2003).

Given the risk of ventricular arrhythmias and sudden death in HCM sufferers, the use of anti-arrhythmic medication may be indicated. The only available medical intervention to prevent sudden death in HCM is amiodarone. However, amiodarone does have a number of side effects (see Chapter 13), so it may not be an acceptable option in children or young adults (McKenna and Behr 2002). The most effective intervention for the prophylaxis of sudden death is the implantation of an implantable cardioverter defibrillator and this should be considered for all patients deemed at high risk of ventricular arrhythmias (McKenna and Behr 2002).

Some surgical and interventional techniques are available to reduce any existing outflow obstruction in patients with HCM. Septal myectomy involves surgically removing a portion of the enlarged myocardium, thereby widening the outflow tract. This operation is usually very effective, with a long-lasting improvement in symptoms, and a surgical mortality rate of less than 3% (Maron et al. 2003). A relatively new technique in the treatment of HOCM is percutaneous alcohol septal ablation. In this procedure, pure alcohol is injected into the coronary artery that supplies the enlarged section of the ventricular septum, causing a limited myocardial infarction. As the infarcted tissue heals, the outflow obstruction reduces in size and thereby eases symptoms (Nishimura et al. 2004). Alcohol septal ablation has been shown to provide symptomatic relief in a large percentage of patients, with fairly low mortality rates (<4%). The most common complication, in up to 30% of patients, is the development of complete heart block requiring permanent pacemaker insertion (Maron et al. 2003). A third technique for the reduction of outflow obstruction is the insertion of a dual chamber pacemaker.

The instigation of a pacing rhythm alters the sequence of ventricular contraction, and this may result in a reduction in outflow obstruction (Chen et al. 2003). However, studies suggest that dual chamber pacing may bring about symptomatic relief in about only 40% of patients (Nishimura et al. 2004). Despite this, the technique does have a place in the treatment of HOCM as an alternative to other surgical procedures.

All patients with HCM will require education and psychological support. Levels of anxiety and depression in HCM patients are significant, often because of uncertainties surrounding the prognosis (Cox et al. 1997). Patients will also need some degree of genetic counselling about their condition (Chen et al. 2003) The genetic nature of HCM means that each child of a HCM sufferer has a 50% chance of inheriting the gene, so the diagnosis has implications for the patient's well-being, and that of the family – presenting a significant challenge to healthcare practitioners (Cruickshank 2004).

RESTRICTIVE CARDIOMYOPATHY

RCM is one of the rarest cardiomyopathies, and is characterised by an increased rigidity in the ventricular wall, not necessarily linked to thickening of the myocardium. A number of different pathophysiological processes can cause this stiffness, including scarring of the heart muscle, or the abnormal deposition of a starch-like substance called amyloid (Chen et al. 2003). Systolic function in RCM may remain near normal, but ventricles are not able to relax properly. Diastolic filling is therefore reduced, leading to systemic and pulmonary venous congestion, coupled with a reduction in cardiac output (Chen et al. 2003).

Signs, symptoms and diagnosis

As with many of the other cardiomyopathies, RCM causes symptoms suggestive of heart failure. Fatigue, breathlessness and peripheral oedema are common, although not specific to RCM (Cruickshank 2004). The chest radiograph often shows a normal size heart, although echocardiography may show enlarged atria and reduced ventricular compliance (Wood and Picard 2004). It is important to try to differentiate between restrictive and constrictive pericarditis (see below), because the two diseases require different treatment strategies. Where available, the most effective diagnostic tools for making this distinction are magnetic resonance imaging (MRI) and myocardial biopsy (Chen et al. 2003).

Clinical management

The aims of treatment for RCM are reduction in venous congestion and prevention of complications. The first of these goals is often achieved through the use of diuretics and vasodilators, although these should be used carefully to avoid excessively reducing ventricular filling pressures (Hoit and Miller 2004). Patients with RCM may develop complications such as atrial fibrillation, thereby increasing their risk of thromboembolic events. If this occurs, anti-arrhythmic agents should be used in an attempt to restore sinus rhythm. If sinus rhythm cannot be maintained or restored, the heart rate should be controlled and the patient anticoagulated with warfarin (Hoit and Miller 2004).

ARRHYTHMOGENIC RIGHT VENTRICULAR CARDIOMYOPATHY

As the name suggests, ARVC is a cardiomyopathy predominantly affecting the right ventricle. It is thought to affect about 1 in 5000 people, and could be responsible for up to 20% of sudden deaths in young people (Francés 2006). ARVC is thought to be the result of a genetic defect that can be transmitted from one generation to the next (Cruickshank 2004). ARVC results in the gradual replacement of normal myocardium in the right ventricle by fatty tissue. The increase in fatty tissue causes weaknesses to form in the right ventricle, eventually leading to dilatation of the chamber (Davies 2000). However, the most serious implication of ARVC is the increased risk of arrhythmias and sudden death.

Signs, symptoms and diagnosis

Sudden death may be the first manifestation of ARVC, particularly in young people (Francés 2006). In those patients who do become symptomatic, common complaints include palpitations resulting from non-fatal arrhythmias, dizziness and shortness of breath (Cruickshank 2004).

Physical examination of patients with ARVC may often fail to detect any major abnormalities, and the chest radiograph may also be normal (Francés 2006). The patient's medical history may include episodes of dizziness and syncope, and there may be a family history of sudden death or diagnosed ARVC (Wood and Picard 2004). Most patients with ARVC will have an abnormal ECG, most commonly displaying T-wave inversion in leads V1–V3. A 24-hour Holter monitor or exercise test may detect the presence of any arrhythmias (Francés 2006). As with most cardiomyopathies, the echocardiogram is a useful diagnostic tool, often demonstrating dilatation or aneurysms present within the right ventricle (Wood and Picard 2004).

Clinical management

Prevention of sudden cardiac death and reduction in symptoms are the priority in managing a patient with ARVC (Cruickshank 2004). Patients who develop symptoms of heart failure should receive standard therapy (e.g. diuretics, ACE inhibitors and digoxin). Sotalol and amiodarone are the anti-arrhythmic agents most commonly used to reduce the risk of ventricular arrhythmias (Francés 2006). For patients at high risk of sudden death, an implantable cardioverter defibrillator may provide the greatest protection. A small number of patients with ARVC may also benefit from radiofrequency ablation of the areas responsible for causing arrhythmias (see Chapter 14) (Francés 2006). Given the genetic nature of the disease, and the possibility of sudden death in young patients, counselling is an important part of the treatment plan. In particular, patients with probable or diagnosed ARVC should be advised not to participate in competitive sports or extreme physical exertion (Francés 2006).

OTHER INFLAMMATORY DISORDERS

PERICARDIAL DISEASE

In health, a thin film of fluid separates the two layers of the pericardial membrane – the visceral and parietal pericardium. However, these layers can become inflamed, a condition known as pericarditis. Although there are many different causes of pericarditis, it will often result either from infection or as a complication of myocardial infarction (MI). Many occurrences of pericarditis are acute in nature, but chronic inflammation of the pericardium is not uncommon, and can last for over 3 months (Maisch et al. 2004). Infectious pericarditis can be either viral or bacterial, and is often secondary to another infection (e.g. influenza, tuberculosis). Infection can also be introduced as a result of chest surgery or penetrating chest trauma. Pericarditis can occur in the days and weeks after an MI. When the condition develops in the first few days after infarction, it is usually a direct result of contact with the inflamed and damaged myocardium. Later-onset MI-related pericarditis, often known as Dressler's syndrome, is thought to be related to the release of antibodies by damaged myocardial cells, and often occurs at least 2 weeks after the MI (Hoit and Faulx 2004).

Patients with acute or chronic pericarditis can develop three potentially serious complications: constrictive pericarditis, pericardial effusion or cardiac tamponade. Constrictive pericarditis is characterised by a chronically inflamed pericardium that becomes progressively stiffened. This loss of flexibility impairs filling of the heart during diastole and reduces cardiac output. Unlike cardiac tamponade, which can develop very quickly, symptoms of constrictive pericarditis increase over a period of months and years. A pericardial effusion is an accumulation of fluid – often excessive amounts of pericardial fluid, exudates or blood. If an effusion develops over time, the pericardium will stretch to accommodate the fluid, allowing as much as 2 litres to build up before symptoms appear (Young and Daniels 2002). However, sudden accumulation of fluid causes the increased pressure in the pericardial sac to press on the heart – a condition called cardiac tamponade. By constricting the heart during diastole, the filling of the heart becomes more difficult and cardiac output begins to fall. If untreated, cardiac tamponade can be fatal.

Signs, symptoms and diagnosis

Patients with acute pericarditis often complain of acute-onset chest pain. This pain is typically sharp in nature, worse on inspiration and relieved slightly by sitting upright. The pain may be associated with shortness of breath, sweating and nausea. The patient may also report feeling generally unwell, and he or she may be pyrexial. In terms of physical findings, the tell-tale sign of acute pericarditis is the presence of a pericardial friction rub, which can be heard when performing auscultation of the chest. A 12-lead ECG may provide some additional evidence for the diagnosis of pericarditis. Widespread, concave (saddle-shaped) ST elevation may be present on the ECG, although it may also be normal in many patients.

The onset of constrictive pericarditis is usually slow. Patients may present with symptoms similar to heart failure, such as shortness of breath and fatigue. A chest radiograph and ECG should be obtained, but may be normal. Echocardiography is a useful investigation for patients with suspected constrictive pericarditis, because it will allow visualisation of the thickened pericardium. Patients with pericardial effusion may present with slow onset of symptoms such as dull chest pain, nausea and vomiting. However, patients with rapid-onset pericardial effusion, leading to cardiac tamponade, will have severe and acute signs and symptoms. This may initially include shortness of breath, restlessness, tachycardia and hypotension. As tamponade develops, the patient's cardiac output will continue to fall, often culminating in a pulseless electrical activity (PEA) cardiac arrest. A pericardial effusion or cardiac tamponade can be definitively diagnosed with an echocardiogram. A chest radiograph may show an enlarged heart, but may also be quite normal.

Clinical management

In patients with uncomplicated acute pericarditis, the priorities are pain relief, reassurance and rest. The most effective analgesics in acute pericarditis are non-steroidal anti-inflammatory drugs (NSAIDs) such as aspirin and ibuprofen. In some patients, treatment with steroids may be necessary. Constrictive pericarditis may respond to medical therapies such as NSAIDs, steroids and antibiotics. Some patients may also gain some temporary relief from symptoms with diuretics. The definitive treatment for constrictive pericarditis is a surgical procedure called pericardiectomy. This operation involves stripping away the diseased pericardium, and carries a mortality risk of 5–15% (Hoit and Faulx 2004).

Patients with a pericardial effusion that causes few symptoms and no haemodynamic instability can be treated medically. Drug therapy such as

NSAIDs or corticosteroids may be useful, and the underlying cause of the effusion should be treated if possible. If the effusion is large enough to cause severe symptoms and a decrease in cardiac output, or if there is any indication of cardiac tamponade developing, the effusion should be drained immediately. Drainage of the effusion is carried out using a procedure called pericardiocentesis, involving insertion of a needle into the pericardial space and aspiration of any fluid. The procedure is carried out under local anaesthetic, and under the guidance of echocardiography or radiography to ensure that the needle enters the pericardial space. Given the likelihood of the effusion returning, a pericardial tap is often inserted to allow constant fluid drainage.

INFECTIVE ENDOCARDITIS

Infective endocarditis (IE) refers to an infection of structures within the heart. Most commonly, the structures affected are either native or prosthetic heart valves, although other foreign bodies such as pacemaker leads can also become diseased (Horstkotte et al. 2004). The infection usually originates elsewhere in the body and travels to the heart via the bloodstream. The infection can be introduced into the bloodstream in a number of different ways. Often, oral bacteria can infiltrate the circulation during dental procedures or even routine care such as tooth brushing. Infection can also be introduced via cardiac surgery or other operations such as tonsillectomy. Intravenous drug users are also at risk of introducing infection into the bloodstream and contracting IE.

Once infection has become established, the patient is at risk of cardiac and non-cardiac complications. If a valve is affected (either native or prosthetic), the areas of infection – known as vegetations – can cause valve dysfunction. IE can also develop into septicaemia or vegetations can become detached from valves and travel into the bloodstream, causing embolic stroke.

Signs, symptoms and diagnosis

Patients will often feel generally unwell for a number of months before a diagnosis of IE is made. They may report general symptoms such as weakness, fatigue and fever. Symptoms such as shortness of breath or chest pain may result from valve dysfunction secondary to infection.

Examination of the patient may reveal that they have a number of non-cardiac symptoms, such as clubbing of the fingers, or small haemorrhages under the nails that look like splinters of wood (Anderson et al. 2004). A heart murmur may be apparent as a result of damage caused to one or more heart valves. Blood cultures should be taken from any patient with suspected IE. Although these may be negative, the vast majority of patients with IE will have positive blood cultures (Anderson et al. 2004). Identification of the bacterial cause of the disease is a crucial step in terms of both diagnosis and treatment. It may be possible to visualise vegetations through the use of echocardiography, so this should be a routine investigation in all patients with suspected IE (Horstkotte et al. 2004). A chest radiograph should be carried out to detect heart failure. Cardiac monitoring and ECGs will not display any changes specific to IE, but will enable detection of any complications (e.g. arrhythmias).

Clinical management

Once a diagnosis has been made, and the bacterium identified, management is initially centred on intravenous antibiotic treatment. The antibiotic used will depend on the bacterium isolated, and treatment regimens will usually last for between 2 and 6 weeks. If the patient does not respond to antibiotic therapy, or if IE recurs despite initial successes, cardiac surgery is often the most effective cure (Eykyn 2001). In some cases, surgical removal of vegetations may be sufficient. However, the level of valve dysfunction caused by the presence of vegetations often results in patients requiring replacement of the affected valve.

Conventionally, patients considered at risk of developing IE, such as those with valve disease or prosthetic heart valves, have been treated with prophylactic antibiotics before certain invasive procedures. In particular, oral and dental procedures have been identified as requiring antibiotic cover for at-risk patients (Danchin et al. 2005). The evidence for the efficacy of antibiotic prophylaxis is fairly limited (Eykyn 2001). However, patients should be educated about the need for antibiotic prophylaxis before invasive procedures, because the recommendation still appears in current IE guidelines (Horstkotte et al. 2004, Danchin et al. 2005)

MYOCARDITIS

As the name suggests, myocarditis is inflammation of the heart muscle. The inflammation usually results from viral infiltration of the myocardium (Pinney and Mancini 2004) as a complication of a respiratory or gastrointestinal infection. Myocarditis can be fatal. Inflammation of the myocardium can cause heart failure and arrhythmias during the acute phase, and result in chronic dilated cardiomyopathy (Chen et al. 2003).

Signs, symptoms and diagnosis

Patients may present with rather general symptoms such as tiredness and fever. However, if the disease has progressed to cause myocardial dysfunction, these may be accompanied by chest pain, shortness of breath and dizziness. In acute myocarditis, these symptoms may develop rapidly, with the patient quickly developing cardiogenic shock.

A number of clinical investigations should be carried out on any patients with suspected myocarditis. The ECG may be abnormal and myocarditis can produce ST-segment elevation similar to that in acute MI. A chest radiograph will show evidence of pulmonary oedema and cardiac enlargement, and echocardiography will detect any ventricular dysfunction. Cardiac enzymes – particularly troponin assays – may be raised in patients with myocarditis. Taking tissue samples from the patient's myocardium and testing for infection can sometimes provide a definitive diagnosis – a procedure called endomyocardial biopsy.

Clinical management

Treatment of the underlying cause of myocarditis is often difficult. If the infection is bacterial, antibiotics are necessary. However, most cases of myocarditis are viral in nature, leaving limited treatment options (Oakley 2000). There is some suggestion that the body's immune response to the viral infection could be a contributory factor in myocarditis. On the basis of this, there has been some suggestion that immunosuppressant therapy such as steroids may be useful. However, there is no conclusive evidence that this is of benefit, and immunosuppressant therapy is not in widespread use for myocarditis (Oakley 2000). In most cases, the priority is to support the patient for the duration of the disease process. At the very least, the patient will need to rest and be closely monitored for deterioration.

Should ventricular dysfunction occur, the patient will initially need pharmacological support such as diuretics and ACE inhibitors. If the patient's condition continues to deteriorate, intra-aortic balloon counterpulsation, or even the temporary use of mechanical circulatory support, may be indicated (Young and Daniels 2002).

CONCLUSION

A wide range of cardiac conditions exist that are not directly linked to coronary heart disease. Valve dysfunction, disorders of the heart muscle, and infections of structures within the heart are all significant causes of mortality and morbidity. By recognising the signs and symptoms of these conditions and utilising effective diagnostic tools, healthcare practitioners can deliver prompt treatment to their patients.

REFERENCES

Anderson J, Sande M, Kartalija M, Muhlestein J (2004) Infective endocarditis. In: Fuster V, Wayne Alexander R, O'Rourke R (eds), *Hurst's The Heart*, 11th edn. New York: McGraw-Hill, pp 2001–34.

Blackburn F, Bookless B (2002) Valve disorders. In: Hatchett R, Thompson D (eds), *Cardiac Nursing. A comprehensive guide.* Edinburgh: Churchill Livingstone, pp 260–86.

Boon N, Bloomfield P (2002) The medical management of valvar heart disease. *Heart* **87**: 395–400.

Carabello B (2002) Aortic stenosis. *New England Journal of Medicine* **346**: 677–82.

Chen Y, Dec W, Lilly L (2003) The cardiomyopathies. In: Lilly L (ed.), *Pathophysiology of Heart Disease*, 3rd edn. Philadelphia: Lippincott, Williams & Wilkins, pp 237–52.

Cox S, O'Donoghue A, McKenna W, Steptoe A (1997) Health related quality of life and psychological wellbeing in patients with hypertrophic cardiomyopathy. *Heart* **78**: 182–7.

Cruickshank S (2004) Cardiomyopathy. *Nursing Standard* **18**(23): 46–52.

Danchin N, Duval X, Leport C (2005) Prophylaxis of infective endocarditis: French recommendations 2002. *Heart* **91**: 715–18.

Davies M (2000) The cardiomyopathies: an overview. *Heart* **83**: 469–74.

Eykyn SJ (2001) Endocarditis: basics. *Heart* **86**: 476–80.

Francés R (2006) Arrhythmogenic right ventricular dysplasia/cardiomyopathy. A review and update. *International Journal of Cardiology* in press.

Hoit B, Faulx M (2004) Diseases of the pericardium. In: Fuster V, Wayne Alexander R, O'Rourke R (eds), *Hurst's The Heart*, 11th edn. New York: McGraw-Hill, pp 1977–2000.

Hoit B, Miller D (2004) Restrictive, obliterative, and infiltrative cardiomyopathies. In: Fuster V, Wayne Alexander R, O'Rourke R (eds), *Hurst's The Heart*, 11th edn. New York: McGraw-Hill, pp 1937–48.

Horstkotte D, Follath F, Gutschik E et al. (2004) Guidelines on prevention, diagnosis and treatment of infective endocarditis. *European Heart Journal* **25**: 267–76.

McKenna W, Behr E (2002) Hypertrophic cardiomyopathy: management, risk stratification, and prevention of sudden death. *Heart* **87**: 169–76.

Maisch B, Seferovic P, Ristic A et al. (2004) Guidelines on the diagnosis and management of pericardial diseases. Executive summary. *European Heart Journal* **25**: 587–610.

Maron B, McKenna W, Danielson G et al. (2003) American College of Cardiology/European Society of Cardiology Clinical Expert Consensus Document on Hypertrophic Cardiomyopathy. *European Heart Journal* **24**: 1965–91.

Nishimura R, Ommen S, Jamil Tajik A (2004) Hypertrophic cardiomyopathy. In: Fuster V, Wayne Alexander R, O'Rourke R (eds), *Hurst's The Heart*, 11th edn. New York: McGraw-Hill, pp 1909–36.

Oakley C (2000) Myocarditis, pericarditis and other pericardial diseases. *Heart* **84**: 449–54.

O'Donoghue A (2002) Cardiomyopathies. In: Hatchett R, Thompson D (eds), *Cardiac Nursing. A comprehensive guide.* Edinburgh: Churchill Livingstone, pp 218–42.

Otto C (2003) Timing of surgery in mitral regurgitation. *Heart* **89**: 100–5.

Pinney S, Mancini D (2004) Myocarditis and specific cardiomyopathies – endocrine disease and alcohol. In: Fuster V, Wayne Alexander R, O'Rourke R (eds), *Hurst's The Heart*, 11th edn. New York: McGraw-Hill, pp 1643–67.

Rahimtoola S (2004) Aortic valve disease. In: Fuster V, Wayne Alexander R, O'Rourke R (eds), *Hurst's The Heart*, 11th edn. New York: McGraw-Hill, pp 1643–67.

Rahimtoola S, Dell'Italia L (2004) Mitral Valve disease. In: Fuster V, Wayne Alexander R, O'Rourke R (eds), *Hurst's The Heart*, 11th edn. New York: McGraw-Hill, pp 1669–93.
Wigle E (2001) The diagnosis of hypertrophic cardiomyopathy. *Heart* **86**: 709–14.
Wood M, Picard M (2004) Utility of echocardiography in the evaluation of individuals with cardiomyopathy. *Heart* **90**: 707–12.
Yachimski P, Lilly L (2003) Valvular Heart Disease. In: Lilly L (ed.), *Pathophysiology of Heart Disease*, 3rd edn. Philadelphia: Lippincott Williams & Wilkins, pp 185–209.
Young J, Daniels L (2002) Pericarditis and myocarditis. In: Hatchett R, Thompson D (eds), *Cardiac Nursing. A comprehensive guide.* Edinburgh: Churchill Livingstone, pp 309–19.

13 Cardiac medications

DAVID BARRETT

Throughout this book, cardiac conditions are discussed and possible treatment strategies outlined. A key element of these treatment strategies is the use of pharmacological agents that affect the function of the heart. This chapter is designed to provide a broad overview of the main drugs used in cardiac care. For each of the drugs discussed, the main actions are explored, and so are its possible indications, contraindications and side effects.

The chapter does not include suggested doses for individual conditions. This partly reflects the introductory nature of the text, and also the fact that specific dosages may alter over time. It is therefore suggested that when dosage information is required, it is taken from an up to date copy of the *British National Formulary* (British Medical Association [BMA] and Royal Pharmaceutical Society of Great Britain [RPSGB] 2005).

ANTIPLATELETS

Platelets are a vital component of the normal clotting mechanism in the body. When injury occurs, platelets become activated and stick first to the area of damage (platelet adhesion) and then to other platelets (platelet aggregation) (Aaronson and Ward 1999). Once activated, platelets also release a number of chemicals that stimulate further platelet aggregation (Martini 2001). The aggregation of platelets at the injury site provides a temporary plug to reduce bleeding while the next element of the haemostatic process (coagulation) can take place. Antiplatelet drugs act in different ways to inhibit the activation and aggregation of platelets, thereby interfering with the clotting process (Ndumele et al. 2003). A number of antiplatelet drugs are used in clinical practice, falling into three main categories: aspirin, ADP-receptor antagonists and glycoprotein IIb/IIIa inhibitors (Knight 2003).

INDICATIONS FOR USE

Aspirin (otherwise known as acetylsalicylic acid) is used to reduce the risk of blood clot formation in a number of cardiovascular disorders. It is indicated

Cardiac Care: An Introduction for Healthcare Professionals. Edited by David Barrett, Mark Gretton and Tom Quinn
© 2006 John Wiley & Sons Ltd

for use in patients with stable angina, to prevent the likelihood of fatal or non-fatal coronary events (Knight 2003). In patients who have had an acute coronary syndromes (ACS), or have undergone cardiac surgery or angioplasty, aspirin should also be taken indefinitely to lower the risks of further cardiac events (White et al. 2005). When administered after an acute cardiac event, an immediate loading dose should be given, either dissolved in water or chewed by the patient, followed by a daily maintenance dose (BMA and RPSGB 2005). Patients with cardiac arrhythmias, particularly atrial fibrillation, are at risk of thrombus formation and embolism and therefore also require treatment with aspirin (Bilal Iqbal et al. 2005).

Clopidogrel is the ADP-receptor antagonist most commonly used in clinical practice. It is often used to prevent future cardiac events in patients who have undergone percutaneous coronary intervention (PCI) (White et al. 2005). Patients undergoing PCI should ideally receive an oral loading dose of clopidogrel before the procedure, and then a maintenance dose for a period of between 2 weeks and 12 months, depending on local guidelines and the type of PCI (Kelly and Steinhubl 2005). Clopidogrel can also be used for the secondary prevention of cardiac events in patients who are unable to tolerate aspirin (Knight 2003).

Glycoprotein IIb/IIIa inhibitors are intravenous antiplatelet agents with a range of clinical indications. Abciximab (ReoPro) is primarily used to reduce the risk of cardiac complications in patients undergoing PCI (BMA and RPSGB 2005). It is also used in patients who have ACS without ST elevation, if the patient is likely to undergo PCI within 24 hours (White et al. 2005). A bolus loading dose of abciximab should be administered, followed by a continuous intravenous infusion for up to 12 hours after the procedure (BMA and RPSGB 2005).

Tirofiban (Aggrastat) and eptifibatide (Integrilin) are two glycoprotein IIb/IIIa inhibitors more commonly used in patients who have ACS without ST elevation, and who are being managed medically (White et al. 2005). It is recommended that one of these agents should be used as part of the initial management of those patients who are considered as being at high risk of myocardial infarction or death (National Institute for Clinical Excellence or NICE 2002).

CAUTIONS, CONTRAINDICATIONS AND SIDE EFFECTS

The greatest risk of administering antiplatelet medication to a patient is bleeding. Patients should therefore be fully assessed and the risks of bleeding complications weighed against the benefits of treatment. These risks are increased if antiplatelet treatment is given in addition to anticoagulant therapy (see below).

Different antiplatelet drugs carry varying risks of bleeding. Aspirin is mostly related to a small risk of gastrointestinal bleeding, although the level of risk can be reduced by taking the drug with food, or using an enteric-coated formulation (White et al. 2005). Clopidogrel administration carries a risk of gastrointestinal and intracranial bleeding, and should therefore not be administered to any patients with evidence of active bleeding (BMA and RPSGB 2005). The greatest risk of haemorrhage is associated with the intravenous glycoprotein IIb/IIIa inhibitors which are contraindicated in patients who have a recent history of active bleeding, major surgery or haemorrhagic stroke (BMA and RPSGB 2005).

Aside from bleeding, specific antiplatelet drugs may cause a number of other side effects, e.g. aspirin and clopidogrel can cause general gastrointestinal upsets, such as indigestion and nausea. Rarely, patients may suffer an allergic reaction to aspirin and it can worsen breathing difficulties in patients with asthma (Ndumele et al. 2003). Patients being treated with glycoprotein IIb/IIIa inhibitors are at risk of developing thrombocytopenia – a reduction in platelet levels (Ndumele et al. 2003). This could exacerbate any bleeding complications and patients should therefore have their platelet levels monitored closely.

ANTICOAGULANTS

Whereas antiplatelet drugs impair the early stages of the clotting process, anticoagulants inhibit the final stage, in which a fibrin clot is formed (Ndumele et al. 2003).

Two main anticoagulants are used in clinical practice: heparin and warfarin. Heparin itself can be split into two main classifications: unfractionated heparin, often given intravenously, and low-molecular-weight heparin (LMWH) given subcutaneously.

INDICATIONS FOR USE

Unfractionated heparin is often administered as an intravenous infusion to patients who have received thrombolytic therapy for acute myocardial infarction. It is also commonly given during PCI procedures as a bolus dose to reduce the risks of cardiac events (White et al. 2005). In many clinical areas, subcutaneous LMWH has become the anticoagulant of choice ahead of unfractionated heparin, largely because of a more predictable anticoagulant effect and fewer side effects (Watson et al. 2002). LMWH, of which Dalteparin and Enoxaparin are examples, can be used to reduce the risk of embolic events in high-risk groups (e.g. those undergoing orthopaedic surgery), and to prevent further cardiac events in patients with ACS (BMA and RPSGB 2005).

Warfarin is an oral medication used for long-term anticoagulation of patients. It is usually targeted at those patients with a history of, or at high-risk of, embolic events – e.g. those with deep vein thrombosis, atrial fibrillation, or mechanical prosthetic heart valves (BMA and RPSGB 2005).

CAUTIONS, CONTRAINDICATIONS AND SIDE EFFECTS

An increased risk of bleeding is the main concern when administering anticoagulant medication, particularly if concurrent antiplatelet therapy is being given. Patients being treated with an intravenous infusion of unfractionated heparin should have the dosage adjusted according to clotting times, and have platelet levels checked every other day (Jowett and Thompson 2003). This will help to reduce the risk of over-anticoagulation and will also detect thrombocytopenia, which occurs in about 10% of patients treated with heparin for more than 5 days (White et al. 2005). Treatment with LMWH can also cause bleeding complications, for which patients must be observed. However, the action of LMWH is more predictable than that of unfractionated heparin, so regular monitoring of clotting times is not necessary (BMA and RPSGB 2005). If patients do show signs of bleeding complications, then heparin therapy should be withdrawn immediately. If this is not sufficient, then the anticoagulant effects of heparin can be counteracted by administration of protamine sulphate (Jowett and Thompson 2003).

Patients on warfarin therapy for long-term anticoagulation are also at risk of bleeding and should be monitored on a regular basis. Monitoring of clotting times in patients taking warfarin is usually through regular measurement of the international normalised ratio (INR). At commencement of warfarin therapy, INR measurement will need to take place on a daily basis to ascertain the appropriate maintenance dose. Once INR measurements have stabilised, then patients will need blood taking every 4–6 weeks to check clotting times (White et al. 2005). If bleeding occurs, then the effects of warfarin can be reversed by the administration of either oral or intravenous vitamin K (BMA and RPSGB 2005).

THROMBOLYTIC AGENTS

When blood clots form, their natural breakdown (fibrinolysis) starts almost immediately (Martini 2001). However, this process can be accelerated by the intravenous administration of thrombolytic drugs. There are a large number of different thrombolytic agents available for use. Streptokinase, one of the earliest thrombolytic drugs, is still in widespread use despite the introduction of a 'second-generation' thrombolytic agent called alteplase (Nordt and Bode 2003). Both streptokinase and alteplase are given via intravenous infusion.

In recent years, 'third-generation' thrombolytic drugs have become more common in clinical practice. These newer agents, of which reteplase and tenecteplase are examples, are given as one or two intravenous bolus doses, making administration quicker and more convenient (Nordt and Bode 2003).

INDICATIONS FOR USE

Thrombolytic agents are utilised for conditions in which thrombi have formed and require dissipating promptly to avoid permanent damage. Non-cardiac indications therefore include deep vein thrombosis and pulmonary embolism (BMA and RPSGB 2005). In cardiac care, thrombolytic agents are primarily used for patients with acute ST-elevation myocardial infarction (MI) as a means of breaking down the blood clot in the coronary artery and restoring blood flow. Early administration of thrombolysis can dramatically reduce mortality rates. However, the longer the delay between symptom onset and treatment with thrombolysis, the less the benefit in terms of mortality (White et al. 2005). Exploration of the use of thrombolysis in MI, including detailed patient criteria, can be found in Chapter 7. It should be noted that thrombolysis should not be used for patients with unstable angina or non-ST-elevation MI, because it has been shown to actually increase mortality in these patients (Betrand et al. 2002).

CAUTIONS, CONTRAINDICATIONS AND SIDE EFFECTS

Bleeding after the administration of thrombolytic therapy is the greatest concern, so patients require close monitoring during and after administration to detect any signs of internal or external haemorrhage. Bleeding may range from fairly minor, such as from intravenous cannulae sites, up to potentially fatal cerebral haemorrhage (Thompson and Webster 2004). To minimise the risk of haemorrhage, a full assessment of the patient must be carried out before administration of thrombolytic therapy. There are many contraindications to treatment, which will vary depending on local guidelines. In general, patients with a recent history of haemorrhage, surgery or trauma should not be treated with thrombolytic therapy (White et al. 2005).

Aside from bleeding complications, patients receiving thrombolytic agents should be observed for hypotension, nausea and vomiting. If the thrombolytic agent successfully restores blood flow through the coronary artery, reperfusion arrhythmias can occur (BMA and RPSGB 2005). Patients receiving streptokinase are at greater risk of allergic reactions than those receiving other thrombolytic agents (White et al. 2005). Crucially, previous treatment with streptokinase causes the body to produce antibodies, reducing the effectiveness of future treatment. Patients who have previously received streptokinase should therefore be treated with another thrombolytic agent (Thompson and Webster 2004).

β Blockers

β receptors are found in the membranes of cells in many organs of the body. The presence of adrenaline (epinephrine) in the body stimulates β receptors, leading to a number of metabolic changes in the target cells. Within the heart, stimulation of specific types of β receptors, called β_1 receptors, will lead to an increase in heart rate and a greater force of cardiac contraction (Martini 2001). β Blockers work by inhibiting the effects of adrenaline on β_1 receptors. This in turn promotes a decrease in heart rate and strength of contraction. These effects result in β blockers decreasing the overall workload of the heart, and thereby reducing the oxygen demand of myocardial cells (Opie and Poole-Wilson 2005). There are many different β blockers available for use, each with slightly different properties and actions. Among the most commonly used agents are atenolol, metoprolol, propranolol, sotalol and carvedilol.

INDICATIONS FOR USE

The therapeutic effects of β blockers on myocardial oxygen demand make them an important therapy in the treatment of hypertension and coronary heart disease (CHD).

In stable angina, use of β blockers will ensure a reduction in episodes of chest pain and greater tolerance for physical activity in the vast majority of patients (Jowett and Thompson 2003). β Blockers are also of use in patients with ACS. There is some evidence that patients with unstable angina and MI may benefit through early treatment with β blockers, either orally or intravenously (Lopez-Sendon et al. 2004a).

After the acute phase of unstable angina or MI, patients who do not have any contraindications should be commenced on a regular regimen of oral β blockers for an indefinite period. Use of a β blocker in patients after an ACS has been demonstrated to reduce mortality and rates of subsequent cardiac events. It is therefore a key element of secondary prevention therapy in patients with CHD (Opie and Poole-Wilson 2005).

Patients with heart failure often have poor left ventricular contraction. It therefore seems unusual that β blockers, with their ability to reduce the strength of cardiac contraction further, would be of any benefit for this client group. However, the use of β blockers in patients with heart failure is now recognised as being extremely beneficial in terms of mortality reduction, and should be part of the standard treatment regimen (Opie and Poole-Wilson 2005). Care should be taken when commencing patients with heart failure on β blocker therapy, with a small initial dose being gradually titrated upwards if the patient does not become hypotensive or bradycardic (Rabin 2003).

In addition to reducing heart rate and the strength of cardiac contraction, all β blockers also have some anti-arrhythmic properties. This particular use of β blockers is discussed below, along with other anti-arrhythmic agents.

CAUTIONS, CONTRAINDICATIONS AND SIDE EFFECTS

Given the therapeutic properties of β blockers, it is hardly surprising that the possible effects of administration are bradycardia and hypotension. As a result of this, one of the most important contraindications to β-blocker use is the presence of symptomatic hypotension (BMA and RPSGB 2005). Usually, the slow heart rate related to β-blocker administration is as a result of a sinus bradycardia. However, β blockers can cause or exacerbate heart block, so they are contraindicated in any patient with second- or third-degree atrioventricular (AV) block, unless a pacemaker has already been inserted (Lopez-Sendon et al. 2004a, BMA and RPSGB 2005).

Possibly the most important non-cardiac contraindication to β-blocker use is a history of asthma (BMA and RPSGB 2005). However, decisions about the administration of β blockers to patients with asthma will depend largely on the severity of lung disease and the potential benefits of β-blocker therapy. In a very small number of patients with asthma, it may be felt necessary to give β blockers, although patients should be monitored closely for any exacerbation of their respiratory disease (BMA and RPSGB 2005).

Some side effects of β blocker use are manifestations of the resulting hypotension and bradycardia (e.g. dizziness). However, patients may experience a range of other side effects such as cold hands and feet, or fatigue (Opie and Poole-Wilson 2005).

Care should be taken when administering β blockers to patients who are taking any other types of drugs with similar actions (i.e. those that reduce blood pressure or reduce heart rate). One particular drug interaction that should be considered is between β blockers and verapamil (see 'Calcium channel blockers' and 'Anti-arrhythmics'). There is a risk of severe hypotension and even cardiac arrest if these drugs are given concurrently, particularly when administered intravenously (BMA and RPSGB 2005). If β blockers are to be stopped for any reason, this should be done gradually. Sudden withdrawal of β blockers can cause an acute increase in myocardial workload, resulting in symptoms such as chest pain and hypertension (Jowett and Thompson 2003).

ANGIOTENSIN-CONVERTING ENZYME INHIBITORS

Long-term blood pressure control in the body is facilitated by the renin–angiotensin system. Angiotensin II, a substance that plays a key role in this system, increases blood pressure in two ways: directly by causing vasoconstriction and indirectly by promoting sodium and water retention. Angiotensin-converting enzyme (ACE) inhibitors decrease the amount of angiotensin II produced and thereby lead to a reduction in blood pressure (McInnes et al. 2004). Many different ACE inhibitors are licensed for use in patients in the UK, with common examples being captopril, lisinopril, ramipril and perindopril.

INDICATIONS FOR USE

The blood pressure-lowering effects of ACE inhibitors make them a useful treatment for three main client groups: those with heart failure, hypertension or a history of MI.

By reducing the amount of angiotensin II produced, ACE inhibitors lessen vasoconstriction and thereby lower the resistance against which the heart has to contract. This allows a failing heart to expel blood more easily, and increases cardiac output (Lopez-Sendon et al. 2004b). This action makes ACE inhibitors the first-line treatment for patients presenting with heart failure (Rabin 2003).

Patients with high blood pressure will often receive treatment with diuretics or β blockers in the early stages of treatment. However, those patients who are not able to tolerate this treatment, or in whom adequate control of blood pressure is not being maintained, should be considered for treatment with ACE inhibitors (BMA and RPSGB 2005).

The third major indication for use of ACE inhibitors is in the secondary prevention of cardiac events in patients with diagnosed CHD. There is evidence that patients with CHD who are treated long-term with ACE inhibitors have fewer subsequent cardiac events and a lower mortality rate than those who are not (Lopez-Sendon et al. 2004b).

CAUTIONS, CONTRAINDICATIONS AND SIDE EFFECTS

Commencement of ACE inhibitor therapy can cause symptomatic hypotension in some patients, so blood pressure monitoring may be required after the initial doses. This is particularly true if the patient is already taking medication that may also lower blood pressure (e.g. diuretics), or has heart failure (BMA and RPSGB 2005). ACE inhibitors can cause acute renal failure, so patients may require close monitoring of urea and electrolyte levels. Monitoring of renal function is especially important in those patients susceptible to kidney failure, such as elderly people or patients with severe heart failure

(Lopez-Sendon et al. 2004b). Renal failure is usually reversible once treatment with ACE inhibitors has stopped (McInnes et al. 2004). Patients who have been diagnosed with bilateral stenosis of the renal arteries should not be given ACE inhibitors because of the increased risk of renal failure (BMA and RPSGB 2005).

Often one of the most troubling symptoms for patients is a dry cough, which occurs in up to 15% of patients (McInnes et al. 2004). The cough can take a number of months to develop after treatment commences, but usually resolves within a few days of ACE inhibitors being withdrawn (Lopez-Sendon et al. 2004b).

ANGIOTENSIN II RECEPTOR BLOCKERS

The action of angiotensin II within the renin–angiotensin system is to increase blood pressure through vasoconstriction and the indirect retention of fluid (see 'ACE inhibitors'). Angiotensin II receptor blockers (ARBs) work by specifically inhibiting the actions of angiotensin II, leading to a reduction in blood pressure (McInnes et al. 2004). Examples of ARBs used in practice are valsartan, losartan and candesartan.

INDICATIONS FOR USE

As with ACE inhibitors, ARBs lower blood pressure by manipulating the renin–angiotensin system. The indications for use are therefore very similar to those for ACE inhibitors. ARBs offer an alternative to ACE inhibitors for patients with hypertension or heart failure, although they are not indicated for secondary prevention in patients with CHD (BMA and RPSGB 2005).

CAUTIONS, CONTRAINDICATIONS AND SIDE EFFECTS

ARBs should be used cautiously in patients with renal artery disease, and they can also cause symptomatic hypotension. In general, however, side effects are far less common than those encountered with ACE inhibitors. Notably, ARB therapy is not associated with a dry cough (McInnes et al. 2004).

CALCIUM CHANNEL BLOCKERS

The movement of calcium into a muscle cell is a key element in the effectiveness of cellular contraction. Within smooth muscle, calcium entry promotes contraction and therefore vasoconstriction. In cardiac cells, increased calcium entry also promotes contraction, but has additional influence on the function of specialist conductive tissue (e.g. sinus node, AV node). The movement of calcium through the membrane and into the cell is facilitated by the presence of calcium channels (Ndumele et al. 2003). By blocking these calcium channels and thereby limiting the amount of calcium entering the cell, calcium channel blockers promote relaxation of smooth muscle (and therefore vasodilatation), reduced strength of cardiac contraction and suppressed electrical conduction (McInnes et al. 2004).

It should be recognised that calcium channel blockers fall into different categories depending on their specific action. The simplest categorisation is that of either dihydropyridines (DHPs) or non-DHPs (Opie 2005). DHPs, which include drugs such as nifedipine and amlodipine, act primarily on smooth muscle to promote vasodilatation in the systemic and coronary circulation. This therefore reduces the resistance against which the heart has to contract, and lowers myocardial oxygen demand. Non-DHPs, such as diltiazem and verapamil, have a greater influence on myocardial contraction and electrical conduction through the heart. They will reduce the strength of contraction, and also reduce the heart rate by inhibiting sinus node activity (Opie 2005).

INDICATIONS FOR USE

All calcium channel blockers, regardless of their specific actions, will lower blood pressure, and decrease myocardial oxygen demand. They are therefore used primarily for patients with hypertension or stable angina. Calcium channel blockers can be used as a first-line therapy for hypertension, and are particularly effective in treating elderly patients (Opie 2005). In patients with angina, calcium channel blockers provide the dual benefit of reducing myocardial oxygen demand (by vasodilatation and/or reduced heart rate and strength of contraction), and possibly increasing oxygen supply through coronary artery dilatation (Ndumele et al. 2003). As the non-DHP calcium channel blockers have an effect on the conduction system of the heart, they are also used as anti-arrhythmic therapy. This use is discussed in depth under 'Anti-arrhythmics'.

CAUTIONS, CONTRAINDICATIONS AND SIDE EFFECTS

The potential adverse effects of calcium channel blockers are largely dependent on the main actions of the agent used. DHPs, in which the primary therapeutic mechanism is systemic vasodilatation, can cause dizziness, flushing and headaches. The reduction in blood pressure can also cause the patient to become tachycardic and experience palpitations (McInnes et al. 2004). As the non-DHPs (diltiazem and verapamil) have an influence on the conduction system and myocardial contraction, their side effects – such as bradycardia and heart blocks – usually reflect this.

None of the calcium channel blockers are recommended for use in patients with heart failure, but left ventricular dysfunction is a particular contraindication for the non-DHPs as a result of their negative effect on contraction (McInnes et al. 2004). Non-DHPs must also be avoided in patients with pre-existing heart block (Opie 2005). The interaction between verapamil and β blockers can have serious cardiovascular consequences and combining the two should be avoided, particularly in the case of intravenous therapy (BMA and RPSGB 2005).

ANTI-ARRHYTHMICS

Anti-arrhythmic agents have traditionally been categorised by their effects on the action potential of cardiac cells (see Chapter 3). Although this type of classification – known as the Vaughan Williams' system – has a number of critics, it is still commonly used to categorise anti-arrhythmic agents. The Vaughan Williams' classification system has four classes of drug, sometimes including a number of subcategories.

Class 1 anti-arrhythmics

Class 1 agents are themselves placed into one of three subcategories – 1A, 1B, or 1C – dependent on their effect on the cardiac action potential. Of all the class 1 agents, lidocaine (previously called lignocaine) is one of the most commonly used.

Class 2 anti-arrhythmics

Class 2 agents – better known as β blockers – are commonly used as anti-arrhythmic agents in addition to their other cardiovascular benefits (see above). Although all β blockers have anti-arrhythmic properties, some are more favoured than others for the treatment of arrhythmias. Examples of those β blockers used to treat arrhythmias are sotalol (which also has strong class 3 anti-arrhythmic properties) and esmolol.

Class 3 anti-arrhythmics

The most widely used class 3 agent is amiodarone, used in the acute and continuing treatment of both ventricular and supraventricular arrhythmias. Similar to all class 3 anti-arrhythmic agents it works by prolonging the action potential of cardiac cells. However, the ability of the drug to treat most tachyarrhythmias is rooted in the fact that it has some properties in common with the other three classes of anti-arrhythmic drugs.

Class 4 anti-arrhythmics

The class 4 agents are more commonly known as calcium channel blockers, and have a number of uses in cardiac disease (see above). In terms of anti-arrhythmic applications, verapamil is the calcium channel blocker most commonly used.

An important anti-arrhythmic agent not accounted for in the Vaughan Williams' classification is the intravenous drug adenosine. Digoxin can be used to modify the heart rate in patients with arrhythmias, and is discussed later in this chapter in the context of inotropic drugs.

INDICATIONS FOR USE

Lidocaine is sometimes used for the suppression and treatment of ventricular arrhythmias, particularly in patients with cardiac disease (Jowett and Thompson 2003).

Of the β blockers with anti-arrhythmic properties, esmolol has the benefit of a short half-life, meaning that its β-blocker effect has ceased within 30 min of administration. It is indicated for use in the acute treatment of narrow complex tachycardia, and is given intravenously (DiMarco et al. 2005). Sotalol can be given intravenously in the emergency treatment of ventricular arrhythmias. However, it tends to be used more commonly in tablet form as prophylaxis for narrow complex tachycardia (particularly atrial fibrillation).

Amiodarone can be administered intravenously as part of the advanced life support protocol for ventricular fibrillation/pulseless ventricular tachycardia. In patients with broad complex tachycardia, intravenous amiodarone is often considered as first-line drug treatment. Amiodarone is also used in the acute and chronic management of narrow complex tachycardia, including atrial fibrillation and flutter (BMA and RPSGB 2005).

Verapamil can be used in the treatment of narrow complex tachycardias, as both an intravenous loading dose and a long-term oral therapy (BMA and RPSGB 2005).

Adenosine is the first-line treatment for patients with narrow complex tachycardia (Blomstrom-Lundqvist et al. 2003). The benefits of using adenosine are that it has a quick onset of action and a short half-life.

CAUTIONS, CONTRAINDICATIONS AND SIDE EFFECTS

It should also be recognised that most anti-arrhythmic agents have the potential to *cause* arrhythmias in some patients (BMA and RPSGB 2005). In addition to a generalised risk of provoking arrhythmias, these agents also have some specific cautions and side effects that need consideration.

Esmolol and sotalol, as with any β blockers, have the potential to cause hypotension and bradycardia, and are generally contraindicated in patients with asthma (see 'β Blockers').

Although amiodarone is a very effective anti-arrhythmic agent, it does have a number of side effects, including nausea, pneumonitis, thyroid dysfunction and liver damage. Some patients on amiodarone also develop corneal microdeposits and a grey discoloration of their skin. Patients taking amiodarone orally for some time should be warned that they may become very sensitive to sunlight. They should be encouraged to avoid exposure to the sun where possible, and to use a sunscreen that protects against UVA and UVB (DiMarco et al. 2005).

If verapamil is used in the management of arrhythmias, the potential interaction with β blockers should be considered (see 'Calcium channel blockers').

DIURETICS

Diuretics influence renal function to increase urine output, and therefore lower the circulating volume of blood. Different types of diuretics have significantly different actions and effects, e.g. loop diuretics such as furosemide and bumetanide are very effective in promoting the excretion of water and electrolytes, and also provoke vasodilatation (Ndumele et al. 2003). Thiazide diuretics (e.g. bendroflumethiazide, metolazone) do not have the potency of loop diuretics, but have a much longer duration of action. Potassium-sparing diuretics (e.g. amiloride, spironolactone), as the name suggests, provide increased excretion of urine while promoting the retention of potassium (Ndumele et al. 2003).

INDICATIONS FOR USE

Diuretics are commonly used in the acute or chronic treatment of heart failure and hypertension. In patients with acute heart failure and pulmonary oedema, intravenous loop diuretics are indicated as a consequence of their ability to induce vasodilatation and promote diuresis quickly (Jowett and Thompson 2003). Loop diuretics are also given in their oral form as long-term therapy for patients with heart failure, sometimes in combination with a thiazide diuretic (Rabin 2003). There is increasing evidence that, when used in heart failure patients, potassium-sparing diuretics can deliver significant improvement in symptoms and reduce mortality rates (Opie and Kaplan 2005). It should be recognised that diuretics in heart failure are used in conjunction with other therapy, notably β blockers and ACE inhibitors. In hypertensive patients, low-dose thiazide diuretics should be instigated as first-line therapy (NICE 2004).

CAUTIONS, CONTRAINDICATIONS AND SIDE EFFECTS

The effects of thiazide and loop diuretics may cause the patient to lose excessive potassium from the bloodstream, causing hypokalaemia (BMA and RPSGB 2005). This may manifest as fatigue and weakness, and leave the patient susceptible to cardiac arrhythmias (Opie and Kaplan 2005). Loop and thiazide diuretics are therefore contraindicated in patients with pre-existing hypokalaemia (BMA and RPSGB 2005). To avoid hypokalaemia, potassium-sparing diuretics can be given either alone or in combination with other diuretics. However, these agents carry the risk of high plasma potassium levels (hyperkalaemia) (Opie and Kaplan 2005). One specific caution is in relation to the administration of intravenous loop diuretics (furosemide, bumetanide). If given too rapidly, these agents can cause damage to the nerve supplying the ears, resulting in hearing impairment (Sanghani and Filer 2002).

ATROPINE

Many episodes of bradycardia are the result of stimulation of the vagus nerve, decreasing the sinus rate or slowing conduction through the AV node. Atropine blocks the effects of the vagus nerve, thereby increasing the heart rate (Ho et al. 2003).

INDICATIONS FOR USE

In terms of cardiac care, intravenous atropine is indicated for patients with symptomatic bradycardia. Intravenous atropine is also given to patients with a cardiac arrest caused by either asystole or pulseless electrical activity (PEA) with a heart rate of less than 60 beats/minute (Jowett and Thompson 2003).

CAUTIONS, CONTRAINDICATIONS AND SIDE EFFECTS

High doses of atropine should be avoided in patients who have recently suffered an MI, because it has been suggested that it may increase the risk of fatal arrhythmias such as ventricular fibrillation (Jowett and Thompson 2003). Given the role of atropine in blocking vagal stimulation, tachycardia is a common side effect for which the patient should be observed.

NITRATES

Nitrates cause dilatation of veins, which reduces the amount of blood returning to the right side of the heart. At higher doses, they also cause dilatation of arteries, reducing the resistance against which the left ventricle has to contract.

These effects result in both a reduction in the workload of the heart and a subsequent decrease in myocardial oxygen demand (Ndumele et al. 2003). Nitrates also dilate coronary arteries, thereby helping to increase myocardial oxygen supply (Bertrand et al. 2002).

Nitrates are available in different preparations, and can be administered through a number of routes. Sublingual nitrates, of which glyceryl trinitrate (GTN) is a common example, are available in tablet or spray form and have a rapid effect when administered under the tongue. GTN is also available for administration through the buccal route, placed between the upper lip and the gum and left to dissolve (BMA and RPSGB 2005). GTN can also be administered via the transdermal route, with a patch applied to the skin for periods of approximately 24 hours. GTN and another nitrate preparation, isosorbide dinitrate, are available in forms that can be given via intravenous infusion for rapid effect. Finally, another nitrate called isosorbide mononitrate is available in tablet form for oral administration, either as a short- or long-acting preparation (BMA and RPSGB 2005).

Nicorandil is a drug properly categorised as a potassium channel activator, but that has nitrate-like properties and a similar mechanism of action. It is available only in tablet form (BMA and RPSGB 2005).

INDICATIONS FOR USE

The reduction in myocardial oxygen demand induced by nitrates makes them an ideal drug for use by patients with angina. In stable angina, patients often administer sublingual or buccal nitrates to relieve episodes of chest pain. There may also be a requirement for patients with stable angina to take regular oral nitrates (Quinn et al. 2002). Nicorandil can be used in patients with stable angina to provide symptom control (BMA and RPSGB 2005). Nitrates are also indicated for use in the management of ACS with intravenous infusion being the route of choice in this context (Bertrand et al. 2002).

Patients with heart failure may benefit from the administration of either intravenous nitrates in acute disease, or oral nitrates for chronic disease management. By reducing the ventricular workload, nitrates can assist a failing heart and reduce pulmonary congestion (Opie and White 2005).

CAUTIONS, CONTRAINDICATIONS AND SIDE EFFECTS

Hypotension can be a common side effect of nitrate therapy, particularly when the drug is administered intravenously. Pre-existing hypotension should therefore be considered a contraindication to treatment with nitrates (BMA and RPSGB 2005). Patients who administer sublingual nitrates in response to the onset of symptoms should be educated about the risk of hypotension and its consequences (e.g. dizziness, fainting) if it is over-administered. It should also be stressed to patients that, if chest pain is not relieved by rest and administration of sublingual nitrates, medical advice should be sought. Common side effects of nitrate administration include headache, dizziness and facial flushing. Patients can develop tolerance to nitrates after long-term use, although this can be lessened by organising dosages to allow for 'nitrate-free' periods (Opie and White 2005).

INOTROPIC DRUGS

Inotropic drugs are those that are used to increase the force with which ventricles contract (Ndumele et al. 2003). A number of different inotropic drugs are used in cardiac care, each with a slightly different mechanism of action. The most commonly used inotropic drugs are digoxin, dopamine, dobutamine, adrenaline (epinephrine) and noradrenaline (norepinephrine).

INDICATIONS FOR USE

Given the ability of inotropic drugs to increase the force of ventricular contraction, the most common indication for use is in patients with acute systolic heart failure or cardiogenic shock (Poole-Wilson and Opie 2005).

For patients with chronic heart failure, digoxin is a relatively weak inotropic agent that may provide some benefit in terms of symptom relief. It is generally used in patients with heart failure who still have symptoms despite a regimen of β blockers, ACE inhibitors and diuretics (Gawlinski and Warner Stevenson 2003). Aside from an increase in the strength of ventricular contraction, digoxin also slows the ventricular rate. This makes digoxin a very useful drug in the control of ventricular rate in patients with persistent atrial fibrillation (Bilal Iqbal et al. 2005). In particular, the dual actions of digoxin make it an ideal agent for patients with heart failure and atrial fibrillation (Jowett and Thompson 2003).

The stronger inotropic drugs – dopamine, dobutamine, adrenaline and noradrenaline – tend to be used for patients with acute systolic dysfunction. They are generally administered as intravenous infusions, with rates titrated according to blood pressure. However, each has slightly different properties and indications.

At low doses, dopamine acts predominantly on the blood supply to the kidneys by dilating renal arterioles. This may enhance renal perfusion, and low-dose dopamine infusions are sometimes used to prevent or treat acute renal failure in patients with systolic dysfunction (Sanghani and Filer 2002). However, there is little clinical evidence to support the effectiveness of low-dose dopamine in protecting renal function, and the use of the drug for this purpose is generally considered to be unjustified (O'Leary and Bihari 2001, Poole-Wilson and Opie 2005).

Dobutamine is usually administered as an intravenous infusion to increase contractility in patients with reduced left ventricular function. Noradrenaline does increase contractility, but also causes systemic vasoconstriction. These two actions make noradrenaline particularly useful in the treatment of patients who are hypotensive as a result of ventricular dysfunction and peripheral vasodilatation (Ndumele et al. 2003).

Adrenaline has two main uses in terms of cardiac care. It can, as with other inotropic agents, be used as an intravenous infusion to enhance ventricular contraction (Poole-Wilson and Opie 2005). However, the predominant use of adrenaline is in the management of cardiac arrest. Aside from inotropic properties, adrenaline also increases the heart rate and causes peripheral vasoconstriction. These properties make adrenaline a key drug in advanced life support, the details of which can be found in Chapter 10.

CAUTIONS, CONTRAINDICATIONS AND SIDE EFFECTS

Patients taking digoxin are at risk of developing digoxin toxicity if levels of the drug in the circulation become too high. Digoxin toxicity can cause signs and symptoms such as nausea and vomiting, confusion and arrhythmias (Poole-Wilson and Opie 2005). Digoxin toxicity should be considered in any patients taking the drug who present with new gastrointestinal, cerebral or cardiac symptoms. This is particularly important for those patients particularly at risk of developing toxicity, such as elderly people or patients with hypokalaemia (BMA and RPSGB 2005). Patients in whom digoxin toxicity is suspected can be diagnosed through the measurement of plasma digoxin levels. Withdrawal of digoxin and correction of hypokalaemia with potassium supplements may be sufficient treatment in most patients (Poole-Wilson and Opie 2005). In severe cases of digoxin toxicity, patients may require treatment with digoxin-specific antibodies (Digibind) (BMA and RPSGB 2005).

One caution regarding increasing contractility with any inotropic drug is that myocardial workload will increase, resulting in a rise in myocardial oxygen demand. In patients with CHD, myocardial ischaemia may therefore result (Ndumele et al. 2003). The use of inotropic agents is also associated with an increased risk of arrhythmias, so close cardiac and haemodynamic monitoring is advisable for patients receiving intravenous inotropic drugs (BMA and RPSGB 2005).

STATINS

Statins provide a pharmacological means to lower total plasma cholesterol levels (Sanghani and Filer 2002). A number of different statin preparations are available for use, including simvastatin, atorvastatin and pravastatin.

INDICATIONS FOR USE

The ability of statins to lower cholesterol levels means that they are widely used in the primary prevention of CHD in high-risk patients – particularly patients with high cholesterol levels (hypercholesterolaemia). Statins should also be used to reduce the incidence of coronary events in patients with diagnosed cardiovascular disease (Department of Health 2000).

CAUTIONS, CONTRAINDICATIONS AND SIDE EFFECTS

Statins are contraindicated in patients with active liver disease. Patients with any history of liver problems, including a high alcohol intake, can be treated cautiously with statins, and liver function should be regularly assessed (BMA and RPSGB 2005).

Patients taking statins may report headaches, nausea, vomiting or diarrhoea. In a small number of patients, potentially serious muscle toxicity can occur. Patients should therefore be encouraged to seek medical advice if they experience unexplained muscle weakness or pain (Gotto and Opie 2005).

CONCLUSION

The practitioner caring for those with cardiac conditions is faced on a daily basis with a cornucopia of different pharmacological agents with which they can treat patients. Each type of drug carries with it different risks and side effects, and its use is underpinned by a rapidly evolving evidence base. Up-to-date knowledge of cardiac medications is therefore crucial if safe and effective care is to be delivered.

REFERENCES

Aaronson P, Ward J (1999) *The Cardiovascular System at a Glance.* Oxford: Blackwell Publishing.

Bertrand M, Simoons M, Fox K et al. (2002) Management of acute coronary syndromes in patients presenting *without* persistent ST-segment elevation. *European Heart Journal* **23**: 1809–40.

Bilal Iqbal M, Taneja A, Lip G, Flather M (2005) Recent developments in atrial fibrillation. *British Medical Journal* **330**: 238–43.

Blomstrom-Lundqvist C, Scheinman M, Aliot E (2003) ACC/AHA/ESC guidelines for the management of patients with supraventricular arrhythmias – executive summary: a report of the American College of Cardiology/American Heart Association Task Force on Practice Guidelines and the European Society of Cardiology Committee for Practice Guidelines. *European Heart Journal* **24**: 1857–97.

British Medical Association and Royal Pharmaceutical Society of Great Britain (2005) *British National Formulary*. London: BMA and RPSGB.

Department of Health (2000) *National Service Framework for Coronary Heart Disease.* London: Department of Health.

DiMarco J, Gersh B, Opie L (2005) Antiarrhythmic drugs and strategies. In: Opie L, Gersh B (eds), *Drugs for the Heart*, 6th edn. Philadelphia: Elsevier Saunders, pp 218–73.

Gawlinski A, Warner Stevenson L (2003) Treatment goals for heart failure patients in critical care. In: Jessup M, McCauley K (eds), *Heart Failure: Providing optimal care*. New York: Futura, pp 83–114.

Gotto A Jr, Opie L (2005) Lipid-lowering and antiatherosclerotic drugs. In: Opie L, Gersh B (eds) *Drugs for the Heart* 6th edn. Philadelphia: Elsevier Saunders, pp 320–48.

Ho J, Stevenson W, Strichartz G, Lilly L (2003) Mechanisms of Cardiac Arrhythmias. In: Lilly L (ed.), *Pathophysiology of Heart Disease*, 3rd edn. Philadelphia: Lippincott, Williams & Wilkins, pp 253–68.

Jowett N, Thompson D (2003) *Comprehensive Coronary Care*, 3rd edn. London: Baillière Tindall.

Kelly R, Steinhubl S (2005) Changing roles of anticoagulant and antiplatelet treatment during percutaneous coronary intervention. *Heart* **91**(suppl III): iii16–19.

Knight C (2003) Antiplatelet treatment in stable coronary artery disease. *Heart* **89**: 1273–8.

Lopez-Sendon J, Swedberg K, McMurray J et al. (2004a) Expert consensus document on β-adrenergic receptor blockers. *European Heart Journal* **25**: 1341–52.

Lopez-Sendon J, Swedberg K, McMurray J et al. (2004b) Expert consensus document on angiotensin converting enzyme inhibitors in cardiovascular disease. *European Heart Journal* **25**: 1454–70.

McInnes G, Curzio J, Kennedy S (2004) Hypertension and antihypertensive therapy. In: Lindsay G, Gaw A (eds), *Coronary Heart Disease Prevention*, 2nd edn. Edinburgh: Churchill Livingstone, pp 371–421.

Martini F (2001) *Fundamentals of Anatomy and Physiology*, 5th edn. NJ: Prentice Hall.

National Institute for Clinical Excellence (2002) *Guidance on the Use of Glycoprotein IIb/IIIa Inhibitors in the Treatment of Acute Coronary Syndromes* London: NICE.

National Institute for Clinical Excellence (2004) *Hypertension. Management of hypertension in adults in primary care* London: NICE.

Ndumele C, Friedberg M, Antman E et al. (2003) Cardiovascular drugs. In: Lilly L (ed.), *Pathophysiology of Heart Disease*, 3rd edn. Philadelphia: Lippincott, Williams & Wilkins, pp 371–421.

Nordt T, Bode C (2003) Thrombolysis: newer thrombolytic agents and their role in clinical medicine. *Heart* **89**: 1358–62.

O'Leary M, Bihari D (2001) Preventing renal failure in the critically ill. *British Medical Journal* **322**: 1437–9.

Opie L (2005) Calcium channel blockers (calcium antagonists). In: Opie L, Gersh B (eds), *Drugs for the Heart*, 6th edn. Philadelphia: Elsevier Saunders, pp 50–79.

Opie L, Kaplan N (2005) Diuretics. In: Opie L, Gersh B (eds), *Drugs for the Heart*, 6th edn. Philadelphia: Elsevier Saunders, pp 80–103.

Opie L, Poole-Wilson P (2005) β-Blocking agents. In: Opie L, Gersh B (eds), *Drugs for the Heart*, 6th edn. Philadelphia: Elsevier Saunders, pp 1–32.

Opie L, White H (2005) Nitrates. In: Opie L, Gersh B (eds), *Drugs for the Heart*, 6th edn. Philadelphia: Elsevier Saunders, pp 33–49.

Poole-Wilson P, Opie L (2005) Digitalis, Acute inotropes, and inotropic dilators. In: Opie L, Gersh B (eds), *Drugs for the Heart*, 6th edn. Philadelphia: Elsevier Saunders, pp 149–83.

Quinn T, Webster R, Hatchett R (2002) Coronary heart disease: angina and acute myocardial infarction. In: Hatchett R, Thompson D (eds), *Cardiac Nursing: A comprehensive guide*. Edinburgh: Churchill Livingstone, pp 151–88.

Rabin D (2003) Pharmacologic management: Achieving target doses and managing interactions. In: Jessup M, McCauley K (eds), *Heart Failure: Providing optimal care*. New York: Futura, pp 165–80.

Sanghani P, Filer L (2002) The pharmacological management of the cardiac patient. In: Hatchett R, Thompson D (eds), *Cardiac Nursing: A comprehensive guide*. Edinburgh: Churchill Livingstone, pp 348–68.

Thompson D, Webster R (2004) *Caring for the Coronary Patient*. Edinburgh: Butterworth Heinemann.

Watson R, Chin B, Lip G (2002) Antithrombotic therapy in acute coronary syndromes. *British Medical Journal* **325**: 1348–51.

White H, Gersh B, Opie L (2005) Antithrombotic agents: platelet inhibitors, anticoagulants, and fibrinolytics. In: Opie L, Gersh B (eds), *Drugs for the Heart*, 6th edn. Philadelphia: Elsevier Saunders, pp 275–319.

14 Interventional cardiology

DAVID BARRETT

Interventional cardiology is an umbrella term that can include a wide range of diagnostic and therapeutic procedures. This chapter discusses those procedures most commonly used, and highlights the main indications for intervention, noteworthy technical aspects and key considerations when caring for patients.

CARDIAC CATHETERISATION AND CORONARY ANGIOGRAPHY

Since its development during the mid-twentieth century, the technique of passing a catheter into the heart and coronary circulation has revolutionised the diagnosis of cardiac disease. By providing a complete picture of a patient's cardiac function, cardiac catheterisation can often give a definitive diagnosis in patients suspected of having valvular disorders, myocardial abnormalities and/or dysfunction, or coronary heart disease (CHD).

Cardiac catheterisation is performed in specialist environments ('laboratories') containing the necessary radiological and medical equipment. Cardiac catheterisation laboratories are now present in most large hospitals, with increasing numbers also found within district general hospitals. The procedures are traditionally performed by cardiologists, with the support of nurses, radiographers and cardiac physiologists. Recent moves to expand the roles of healthcare practitioners have led to some diagnostic procedures being performed without a doctor present.

A rapid expansion in cardiac catheterisation facilities within the UK, particularly in England, has been seen since the publication of the National Service Framework (NSF) for CHD (Department of Health or DH 2000). Since 2002, 87 new cardiac catheterisation laboratories either have opened or are due to open by 2007 (DH 2005). Largely as a result of this expansion, the total number of diagnostic procedures in the UK now exceeds 200000 annually (British Cardiovascular Intervention Society or BCIS 2005).

Cardiac Care: An Introduction for Healthcare Professionals. Edited by David Barrett, Mark Gretton and Tom Quinn
© 2006 John Wiley & Sons Ltd

METHODS

Access to the heart is achieved via a peripheral blood vessel. After cannulation of the blood vessel with a needle, a sheath is inserted to prevent blood loss during the procedure, while still allowing cardiac catheters to be passed. The patient is usually awake during the procedure, with local anaesthetic given at the catheter access point.

Catheterisation of the right side of the heart is sometimes carried out to allow for assessment of right atrial or ventricular pressures, pulmonary or tricuspid valve function, or structural abnormalities such as septal defects. To achieve access to the right side of the heart, the catheter is usually passed through the femoral vein and up into the heart.

More commonly, access is required to the left side of the heart and coronary circulation. In most cases, the femoral artery is used as the point of access through which the aorta and left side of the heart can be approached, although the use of a radial artery is becoming increasingly popular. Once in the arterial system, the catheter is passed up into the aorta. At this point, the operator can pass the catheter either into the coronary circulation or through the aortic valve and into the left ventricle. To facilitate this, many different types of catheter are produced, each with specially shaped ends to ease passage into the different areas of the coronary anatomy.

Once correctly positioned, pressure readings can be taken through the end of the catheter. Radio-opaque dye is also injected through the catheter at the same time as moving radiological images are recorded. Where the left ventricle has been catheterised, this allows for visualisation of the function of the chamber and the detection of any valvular problems such as aortic or mitral regurgitation. In coronary angiography, where the left or right coronary circulation is catheterised, the passage of dye through each artery allows the operator to detect any atherosclerotic plaques or thrombi.

CARE OF THE PATIENT

Before elective cardiac catheterisation, patients need a period of fasting, usually of no less than 6 hours (Busch et al. 2000). Patients normally taking warfarin should ideally omit three doses before the procedure to reduce the risks of bleeding complications, although other antiplatelet and anticoagulant therapy (such as aspirin or heparin) is usually continued (Bashore et al. 2001). Some patients may have allergic reactions to the radio-opaque dye used in cardiac catheterisation. Any reactions that occurred in previous procedures should therefore be documented during the pre-procedure assessment, and patients at risk of further allergic responses may benefit from pre-treatment with steroids. There is some evidence that the dye can interact with the drug metformin – commonly used by patients with diabetes – and cause renal dysfunction. It is therefore recommended that metformin be omitted on the morning of the procedure, and for 48 hours after completion of the procedure (Bashore et al. 2001).

When the procedure is carried out electively, patients are usually treated as day cases. Complication rates are low, with the chances of death approximately 1 in 1400 (Grech 2004a, West et al. 2005). The chances of complications do increase depending on the patient's age, general health and severity of CHD, so individual assessment should always be made before obtaining informed consent.

Before the procedure, the patient should be informed of the possibility of some angina-like discomfort during coronary angiography. He or she should also be aware that, if ventricular angiography is performed, the large amount of dye injected could result in a short-lived hot flush, and the mistaken feeling that he or she has been incontinent of urine.

At the end of a diagnostic procedure, the access sheath is usually removed, and haemostasis achieved using manual pressure. Access site complications such as haemorrhage or haematoma are the most common problems encountered by patients after diagnostic coronary catheterisation. Although major vascular complications (such as damage to an artery requiring surgical repair) may occur in only about 1 in 500 procedures (Grech 2004a), minor vascular complications such as haematoma are evident in as many as 1 in 5 patients (West et al. 2005). For this reason, close observation of the access site is vital when caring for the patient post-procedure. In the case of femoral arterial access, patients should remain flat in bed for at least 1 hour and on bed rest for at least 2.5 hours to minimise the chance of post-procedure vascular complications (Pollard et al. 2003). Where radial access has been used, patients may mobilise much sooner. If recovery is uncomplicated, patients can be discharged a few hours after the procedure. Where possible, the findings of the study, and a proposed plan of care, should be provided to the patient before discharge home.

ELECTROPHYSIOLOGICAL STUDIES AND RADIOFREQUENCY ABLATION

Whereas cardiac catheterisation and coronary angiography can identify structural abnormalities and coronary artery disease, electrophysiological studies (EPS) offer insight into the electrical activity within the heart. For this reason, EPS are often indicated as a means of investigating patients with a history of palpitations and faints, or patients with documented arrhythmias (Kaye 2004).

Many aspects of EPS, such as patient preparation and aftercare, are similar to those for cardiac catheterisation. However, the procedure is technically much more complex. A number of catheters tipped with electrodes are passed into the heart percutaneously. Measurements are taken via the electrodes, which provide information about the function of the conduction system of the heart during rest. However, more useful information can often be gathered by inducing arrhythmias through the use of pacing wires. Provocation of arrhythmias can allow the mapping of abnormal electrical activity, ideally allowing the point of origin to be ascertained.

If studies do result in the identification of abnormal pathways that sustain arrhythmias, a treatment known as radiofrequency ablation can be used. A further catheter tipped with electrodes is passed percutaneously into the heart and positioned by the abnormal area of myocardium. Once in place, high-frequency electrical current – known as radiofrequency energy – is passed through the electrodes, thereby destroying the point of arrhythmia activation (Blancher and Main 2000).

As with cardiac catheterisation and percutaneous coronary intervention (PCI – see below), the care of the patient after EPSs or radiofrequency ablation is centred on reducing access site complications and early detection and management of cardiac complications. Patients will need a number of hours on bed rest if the femoral vein and/or artery has been used for catheter access. Depending on the type of arrhythmia being treated, patients may be at risk of developing complete heart block as a result of ablation. In particular, patients undergoing ablation to treat junctional re-entrant tachycardia have a 1–2% risk of requiring permanent pacemaker insertion as a result of the development of heart block (Kaye 2004).

PERCUTANEOUS CORONARY INTERVENTION

PCI was first carried out on a human in 1977. Since then, the technology has developed and techniques enhanced to such a degree that PCI has overtaken coronary artery bypass (CAB) as the most commonly used intervention for patients with CHD. In the UK, 63 000 PCI procedures were carried out in 2004, almost double the number carried out in 2000 (BCIS 2005). PCI can be performed electively to reduce symptoms in patients with stable angina (see Chapter 6). Increasingly, PCI is used in the emergency treatment of acute coronary syndromes, as either an adjunct or an alternative to first-line pharmacological therapy (see Chapter 7).

METHODS

PCI involves taking the fundamental principles of coronary angiography and building on them. In most cases, catheters with a deflated balloon on the end are passed into a diseased coronary artery and positioned within an atherosclerotic plaque. Once correctly positioned, the balloon is filled at a high pressure with a mixture of radio-opaque dye and heparin. This 'squashes' the area of plaque against the artery wall, enlarging the lumen at the point of balloon inflation. When used alone, the process of dilating the artery through balloon inflation is known as percutaneous transluminal coronary angioplasty

(PTCA). Although often effective, PTCA can be followed by acute or chronic re-occlusion of the treated area, or be complicated by dissection of the artery wall.

To optimise treatment and reduce re-occlusion rates, metal stents are almost always inserted at the point of treatment after PTCA. Stents are mounted on PTCA balloons and passed into the diseased area. When the balloon is inflated, the stent is expanded and pressed against the artery wall. On deflation of the balloon, the stent remains in position, acting as 'scaffolding' for the artery wall. The development of stents as an adjunct to PTCA has decreased re-occlusion and mortality rates significantly. As technology has progressed, stents have been developed that allow for insertion in small arterial branches and at junction points in the coronary circulation. This flexibility in their use has led to PTCA and stenting becoming the predominant type of PCI utilised in clinical practice. The ability to stent multiple lesions has also led to more patients becoming suitable for PCI in preference to CAB. Recently, work has been carried out on stents to try to reduce re-occlusion rates further. Radiation treatment of stents has been shown to be slightly beneficial, but the most promising development is that of drug-eluting stents (DES). After insertion, these slowly release pharmacological agents that inhibit cell proliferation. Use of a DES in preference to a bare metal stent has been shown to reduce re-occlusion rates significantly, and DES are now used in about 50% of PCI cases in the UK (BCIS 2005).

Although PCI is predominantly carried out through PTCA and stent implantation, some other devices can be used. Coronary atherectomy can be carried out through the insertion of a specialist catheter with a small drill on the end. Once in position next to the plaque, the drill rotates at up to 200 000 rev/minute (rpm) and cuts away at the lesion (Windecker and Meier 2000).

PHARMACOLOGICAL ADJUNCTS

PCI procedures, whether inflating a balloon, deploying a stent or using a drill, all cause damage to the atherosclerotic plaque and coronary artery wall. This therefore puts patients having PCI at significant risk of developing thrombi in their coronary arteries as a response to injury, resulting in myocardial infarction (MI) (Philipp and Grech 2004). To reduce the risk of thrombus formation, patients undergoing PCI are treated with a cocktail of anticoagulant and antiplatelet agents. Although indications for drugs in the context of PCI are discussed in this chapter, the details of side effects and contraindications can be found in Chapter 13.

Heparin should be given to all patients undergoing PCI. Unfractionated heparin remains the most commonly used form in PCI, although there are a number of studies evaluating the safety and effectiveness of low-molecular-weight heparin (LMWH) in this context (Kelly and Steinhubl 2005).

Of the antiplatelet therapies available, aspirin reduces the risk of acute coronary artery closure in PCI by up to 75% (Philipp and Grech 2004). Patients who are not already on aspirin before PCI should be given a loading dose before the procedure, and remain on a daily maintenance dose indefinitely, unless they have a known allergy (Silber et al. 2005).

Recent studies have demonstrated that treatment with the oral antiplatelet agent clopidogrel in combination with aspirin reduces the likelihood of thrombus formation after stent insertion (Silber et al. 2005). Ideally patients should be pre-treated with a loading dose of 300 mg clopidogrel at least 6 hours before any PCI procedure (Kelly and Steinhubl 2005). After stent insertion, patients will remain on a maintenance dose of clopidogrel for a period of at least 3–4 weeks, although there is increasing evidence that longer administration periods of up to a year are clinically beneficial (Philipp and Grech 2004).

Glycoprotein (GP) IIb/IIIa inhibitors are a class of antiplatelet agents that can reduce the likelihood of major adverse cardiac events (MACE) during or after PCI (Kelly and Steinhubl 2005). As a result of the clinical effectiveness of GP IIb/IIIa inhibitors, they are recommended for use in high-risk elective PCI, or in all patients who require emergency PCI to manage an acute coronary syndrome (Silber et al. 2005). Three intravenous GP IIb/IIIa preparations are currently used within the UK: abciximab (ReoPRo), eptifibatide (Integrilin) and tirofiban (Aggrastat). Studies in patients undergoing PCI suggest that, of these three, abciximab provides the greatest clinical benefit and should be the agent of choice (Dawkins et al. 2005). Many patients will have a GP IIb/IIIa inhibitor started in the catheterisation laboratory during PCI, continuing for about 12–16 hours after completion of the procedure (Silber et al. 2005).

COMPLICATIONS

PCI carries a much higher rate of mortality and morbidity than diagnostic cardiac catheterisation or coronary angiography, although the procedure is now much safer than in earlier years. Overall mortality rates in 2004 were 0.56%, although – as might be expected – rates are much higher in emergency and high-risk procedures (BCIS 2005). Overall, PCI also carries a small risk of MI (0.3%), or the need for emergency CAB (0.21%) or emergency repeat PCI (0.3%) (BCIS 2005). Patients undergoing PCI also have a 1 in 300 risk of having a haemorrhagic or non-haemorrhagic cerebrovascular accident (CVA) during or after the procedure (Dukkipati et al. 2004).

In addition to the increased risk of MACE in patients undergoing PCI, the pharmacological adjuncts discussed above – anticoagulant and antiplatelet agents – greatly increase the risk of access point bleeding complications. It has been suggested that up to 8% of patients undergoing PCI through the femoral artery have some type of vascular complication (Archbold et al. 2004). However, the rate of vascular complications is greatly reduced when the radial artery is the point of access, and this approach is now adopted in about 10% of PCI procedures (BCIS 2005).

Given the higher potential for complications, PCI is traditionally carried out in a cardiac catheterisation laboratory that has access to cardiac surgery facilities. Although these facilities do not necessarily need to be within the same hospital as that in which PCI takes place, processes should be in place to ensure that bypass can be established within 90 minutes of referral for emergency surgery (Dawkins et al. 2005).

PERCUTANEOUS VALVULAR AND SEPTAL DEFECT REPAIR

Valvular disease is discussed in Chapter 12, with surgical management explored in Chapter 15. For patients with valve disease, there are a number of percutaneous procedures that can provide alternatives to purely medical or surgical management.

When valves are stenotic, a procedure known as a valvuloplasty can be used. This procedure is relatively uncommon, with just 215 valvuloplasty procedures carried out in the UK in 2004, most of which were to treat mitral stenosis (BCIS 2005). The technique for valvuloplasty involves passing a catheter into the heart via a large peripheral blood vessel and through the stenotic valve under radiological guidance. In mitral valvuloplasty, the most common technique is to use the femoral vein as access, and then access the mitral valve by puncturing the atrial septum and passing the catheter into the left atrium (Vahanian 2001). In most procedures, the catheter has a balloon on the end, which is deflated to allow passage through the valve. Once in position, the balloon is inflated, thereby dilating the stenotic valve.

Valvuloplasty does carry a number of risks. Mitral valvuloplasty has a mortality rate of about 1%, and can cause severe mitral regurgitation in 2% of patients (Grech 2004b). In addition, re-stenosis of the valve occurs in up to 40% of patients within 8 years, requiring repeat valvuloplasty (Grech 2004b). The risks of aortic valvuloplasty are much higher than those associated with mitral valve procedures, with up to a quarter of patients having serious complications, and a hospital mortality rate reportedly of between 3.5% and 13.5% (Vahanian and Palacios 2004). The high complication rate, coupled with a lack of long-term benefits, make aortic valvuloplasty of use only for adults in whom surgery is unsuitable (National Institute for Clinical Excellence or NICE 2004). It should be noted, however, that in children, balloon aortic valvuloplasty has greater effectiveness than in adults and therefore remains the usual treatment choice for paediatric aortic stenosis (Walsh 2004).

Although valve replacement is carried out only surgically at present, work is ongoing in developing percutaneous techniques for aortic and mitral valve replacement. The first percutaneous aortic valve replacement was carried out in 2002, and the technique may become a valuable option for patients with severe valve disease who are considered unsuitable for surgery (Vahanian and Palacios 2004).

Septal defects usually either occur as a result of congenital heart disease or may present as a complication of acute MI. Atrial septal defects can be closed percutaneously by passing a specialist catheter through the femoral vein, and inserting a closure device into the defect (Piéchaud 2004). A similar technique can be used for closure of a patent foramen ovale (PFO) and, in total, over 800 of these closure procedures were carried out in the UK in 2004 (BCIS 2005). Percutaneous closure of ventricular septal defects is much rarer and more technically challenging. Although a number of percutaneous ventricular defect closures have been carried out to good effect, it is not yet clear whether this procedure provides a safe alternative to surgical closure, or simply an option for patients unsuitable for surgery (Piéchaud 2004).

PACEMAKERS

Cardiac pacemakers are devices designed to provide an artificial electrical stimulus to cardiac muscle cells, thereby prompting depolarisation and contraction (Barnett 2002). Pacemakers can broadly be categorised according to whether they are designed for temporary or permanent use by the patient. In addition, temporary pacemakers can be either internal or external. This chapter reviews the different forms of pacemaker, taking account of the indications for use, procedure for insertion and patient care.

INDICATIONS FOR PACING

Common indications for pacing relate to the presence of potentially dangerous bradyarrhythmias such as second-degree atrioventricular block Mobitz type II, or third-degree (complete) heart block (Vijayaraman and Ellenbogen 2004) (see Chapter 9). Pacing can also be used as a therapy in the cessation of tachycardia, a procedure known as overdrive pacing, or sometimes as anti-tachycardia pacing (ATP). There is increasing evidence that some patients with heart failure may benefit from having pacemakers inserted that simultaneously pace both ventricles. This approach, known as biventricular pacing, is thought to improve haemodynamic status and exercise tolerance by resynchronising ventricular contraction (Bleasdale and Frenneaux 2004).

PRINCIPLES OF PACING

In health, the conduction system of the heart acts to transmit a wave of depolarisation throughout the myocardium, thereby stimulating contraction. A number of diseases and defects can cause the conduction system to become dysfunctional, or to fail altogether. Cardiac pacemakers can benefit patients with conduction defects by providing an artificial stimulus that prompts myocardial depolarisation. It is possible to pace atria, ventricles or both, depending on the needs of the patient.

To provide an artificial electrical stimulus, a cardiac pacemaker requires a number of different components. The pulse generator controls the rate and strength of the stimulus, and also includes a circuit that enables sensing of the patient's intrinsic cardiac activity. This ability to sense cardiac activity is a key part of the pacemaker system, because it enables the pacemaker to deliver a stimulus only when necessary. If a pacemaker delivers electrical stimuli at a fixed rate, regardless of the patient's own cardiac activity, an artificial impulse could be delivered during the repolarisation phase of the patient's own electrical impulse, potentially causing ventricular fibrillation (Jacobson and Gerity 2000). In demand pacing, the pulse generator senses intrinsic cardiac activity and withholds the delivery of an artificial stimulus as appropriate – thereby reducing the likelihood of ventricular fibrillation.

The rate and strength of the electrical stimuli produced by the pulse generator can be adjusted to adapt to changing patient needs. Selection of the correct strength of electrical stimuli is particularly important, because the required energy may alter with time. The strength of stimuli required to prompt myocardial depolarisation – referred to as capture – is known as the threshold. If the threshold increases, which can occur over time, the output of the pacemaker must be increased to ensure consistent capture (Jacobson and Gerity 2000).

In addition to the pulse generator, all pacemakers require at least one pacing lead, which is a wire connecting the pulse generator to the myocardium. Leads will vary depending on the type of pacemaker system being used. In patients with a temporary pacemaker (discussed below), additional cables are often required to connect the pulse generator to the pacing lead(s).

Pacemakers are classified depending on a number of different functions. For most pacemakers, a three-letter system defines their main characteristics. The first letter represents the chambers that are being paced, the second letter relates to the chambers in which intrinsic cardiac activity is sensed, and the third letter describes the pacemaker's response to sensing the patient's own electric impulse. For example, a pacemaker that paces only the ventricle (V), senses only in the ventricle (V) and inhibits (I) the next artificial stimulus in response to sensing intrinsic electrical activity would be referred to as a VVI pacemaker.

More complex pacemakers with two pacing leads are able to pace and sense in the right atrium and ventricle, and are referred to as dual chamber systems. In an attempt to mimic normal physiological processes, dual chamber pacemakers have a dual response to sensing inherent electrical activity. If atrial activity is sensed, but no ventricular activation follows, an artificial stimulus is provided via the ventricular lead. If a ventricular lead senses intrinsic ventricular activity, the artificial stimulus is inhibited. The dual chamber pacing and sensing capability, coupled with a dual response to sensing, results in these pacemakers often being categorised as DDD pacemakers (Vijayaraman and Ellenbogen 2004).

TEMPORARY PACING

Temporary pacing is commonly used as a short-term intervention in the management of bradycardic patients who are haemodynamically compromised or otherwise at high risk of developing a dangerously slow heart rate. There are three main routes through which a patient can be paced: transvenous, epicardial and transcutaneous (external).

Transvenous pacing

This is carried out by passing the lead into a vein (usually a subclavian, internal jugular or femoral vein) under local anaesthetic (Betts 2003). The lead is passed into the right side of the heart under radiological guidance and manipulated so that the end of the lead is placed against the myocardium. As a result of the potential risk of pacing leads becoming displaced over time, some leads now include fixation devices such as screws that improve the reliability of transvenous pacing (Gammage 2000). Once in place, the leads are attached to a pulse generator, the pacing threshold is tested and, if acceptable, the leads are secured to the skin at the entry point to reduce movement. Patients with transvenous pacing leads *in situ* should be monitored closely for any signs of lead displacement or infection. Threshold testing should be carried out daily, continuous cardiac monitoring should be maintained to detect arrhythmias and the importance of not spilling water on the pulse generator should be reinforced (Barnett 2002). The removal of transvenous pacing wires should ideally be carried out while cardiac monitoring is still ongoing, because movement of the lead can provoke arrhythmias. Patients in whom either the subclavian or jugular route was used should be laid flat with their head slightly down to reduce the risk of air embolism, and the wound site covered with an air-occlusive dressing after removal (Barnett 2002).

Epicardial pacing

This is usually used in cardiac surgery as prophylaxis against any postoperative bradyarrhythmias (see Chapter 15). During surgery, pacing leads are attached to the outside wall of the myocardium and then brought out through the skin. When epicardial wires are removed, either deliberately or through accidental dislodgement, there is some risk of bleeding and cardiac tamponade. Patients should therefore be monitored closely after removal for any signs of haemodynamic instability (Inwood 2002).

Transcutaneous pacing

This can be used as a non-invasive and rapidly initiated form of pacing in emergency situations, including outside a hospital in selected cases by appropriately trained ambulance personnel. Two large adhesive pacing electrodes are placed on the patient, with one on the chest over the heart and the other on the back just below the left shoulder blade (Barnett 2002). The electrodes are connected to a pulse generator, which is usually a defibrillator with pacing capability. The electrical stimulus passes through the chest and heart, thereby achieving capture. Given the distance that the stimulus has to travel to reach the heart, a high level of current is required. This can cause distress and pain to the patient, so some sedation may be required. The difficulty that can be experienced in achieving and maintaining capture, coupled with the level of patient discomfort, means that transcutaneous pacing should be used only as an emergency measure until transvenous pacing can be initiated (Jacobson and Gerity 2000).

PERMANENT PACING

A permanent pacemaker is one in which the entire mechanism – pulse generator and pacing leads – is implanted within the patient. This procedure is carried out under local anaesthetic, using a strict aseptic technique. The pacing leads are inserted first and an appropriate threshold achieved. The pulse generator is then attached and placed in a subcutaneous pocket, usually positioned in the upper pectoral region (Vijayaraman and Ellenbogen 2004). Rates of permanent pacemaker insertion continue to rise year on year, with 30 000 systems inserted in the UK in 2004 (Cunningham 2005). Once implanted, a permanent pacemaker system can be re-programmed externally by cardiac physiologists, using radiofrequency devices. The batteries within permanent systems can last up to 12 years, after which time the pulse generator will require replacement (Barnett 2002).

A number of early and late complications can occur after permanent pacemaker implantation. Dislodgement of the pacing lead(s) can occur soon after implantation in about 2.5% of patients (Pavia and Wilkoff 2001). In the immediate postoperative period, patients should be closely observed for external bleeding or haematoma at the wound site, which occurs in just under 5% of cases (Wiegand et al. 2004). Although many haematomas will resolve without invasive treatment, about 1% of patients may require further surgery to manage bleeding complications (Wiegand et al. 2004). Other potential complications include pneumothorax as a result of accidental lung injury, cardiac tamponade caused by perforation of the atrial or ventricular wall, and arrhythmias resulting from myocardial irritation by pacing leads (Pavia and Wilkoff 2001). Patients should therefore be monitored for these rare, but potentially life-threatening, early complications during the first few hours after the procedure. Pre-discharge checks should always include a chest X-ray and pacemaker check to ensure correct positioning and function (Barnett 2002).

Longer-term complications of permanent pacemaker implantation tend to be related to the pocket in which the pulse generator is placed within the patient's body. Over time, the pulse generator can gradually erode the subcutaneous tissue around it, and on occasions this can result in the skin above the pacemaker being eroded. Infection of the pacemaker is a serious problem often associated with erosion of surrounding tissue. Patients undergoing pacemaker insertion are therefore routinely given antibiotics after the procedure and, in some centres, antibiotic fluids are used to irrigate the pocket during implantation (Vijayaraman and Ellenbogen 2004). Post-procedure care must include regular temperature monitoring to detect systemic infection, and patients should be educated to recognise any signs of infection (e.g. inflammation, fever) after discharge. Patients having a ventricular pacemaker inserted should also be made aware of the risk of 'pacemaker syndrome'. This condition, affecting up to 7% of patients, is caused by the loss of synchronisation between atrial and ventricular contraction (Vijayaraman and Ellenbogen 2004). The symptoms of pacemaker syndrome are varied, but patients predominantly report feeling tired, breathless and dizzy.

Routine follow-up of patients who have had a permanent pacemaker inserted is important to allow evaluation of key issues such as battery life and pacing threshold. Rates of follow-up will depend on patient history and clinical preference. However, as a broad guideline, patients will attend a pacemaker clinic twice in the first 6 months after implantation, and then every 6–12months subsequently (Gregoratos et al. 2002).

Implantation of a permanent pacemaker will require some lifestyle adjustment by the patient. In the short term, patients will be advised to refrain from excessive physical activity to allow the wound to heal properly. Within the UK, patients must refrain from driving for at least 1 week after pacemaker insertion (Barnett 2002). A number of sources of electromagnetic interference, in both the clinical setting and everyday life, can affect pacemaker function. Clinically, procedures such as defibrillation or electrocautery can stop pacemaker function, and pacemaker checks must be carried out subsequent to exposure to sources of electric energy. Magnetic resonance imaging (MRI) can cause a potentially dangerous malfunction within the pulse generator, and should be avoided if possible in patients with a pacemaker (Vijayaraman and Ellenbogen 2004). In the wider world, devices such as mobile phones and airport/shop security scanners can cause electromagnetic interference that may affect pacemaker function. Mobile phones should not be kept in a pocket directly over the pacemaker and, where possible, should be held to the ear on the opposite side of the body to that in which the pulse generator resides. Patients with pacemakers should be encouraged to walk briskly through security scanners (Barnett 2002), taking care to alert security staff about the existence of a pacemaker to avoid causing undue anxiety.

IMPLANTABLE CARDIOVERTER DEFIBRILLATORS

Implantable cardioverter defibrillators (ICDs) are devices capable of detecting and treating a range of potentially fatal arrhythmias. The ability of ICDs to sense rhythm abnormalities, provide pacing in episodes of bradycardia and deliver cardioversion/defibrillation shocks for tachyarrhythmia makes them an increasingly popular method of preventing sudden cardiac death. As with permanent pacemakers (see above), ICDs incorporate a pulse generator attached to leads that sit against the myocardium within the right ventricle and, on occasions, the right atrium (Houghton and Kaye 2004). The electrodes are able to sense, pace (in response to either bradycardia or tachycardia) and deliver defibrillatory shocks as required.

ICDs are indicated in patients at risk of sudden cardiac death, and can be used in either a primary or secondary prevention role. Patients requiring primary prevention are those with no previous history of sustained ventricular arrhythmias, but with risk factors that suggest that they are susceptible to sudden cardiac death (National Institute for Health and Clinical Excellence or NICE 2006). These risk factors include MI resulting in left ventricular dysfunction and episodes of ventricular tachycardia (VT), or any genetic condition that carries a high risk of sudden cardiac death. Secondary prevention use is indicated in those patients with a history of sustained VT, or cardiac arrest caused by ventricular fibrillation (VF) or VT, where there is no treatable cause (NICE 2006). Recognition of the clinical effectiveness of ICDs in preventing sudden cardiac death has led to an increase in their use. In the UK, the number of ICDs implanted has grown tenfold in a decade, from 224 in 1994 to 2337 in 2004 (Cunningham 2005).

The technicalities of implanting an ICD are similar to those involved with a permanent pacemaker (see above). The most significant additional element of the procedure is for the defibrillatory threshold to be checked by inducing VF/VT and ensuring that the defibrillator efficiently senses the arrhythmia and delivers an appropriate shock, thereby re-establishing sinus rhythm. Post-procedure care also shares a number of similarities with permanent pacemaker insertion, and focuses on the detection and prevention of complications such as bleeding, infection, lead dislodgement and structural damage to the heart or blood vessels (James 2002). Infection is a particularly serious risk after ICD implantation, with about 0.5% of patients developing an infection that necessitates removal of the device (Alter et al. 2005). For this reason, a course of prophylactic antibiotics is an important element of post-procedure treatment (James 2002).

Structured aftercare of patients in the months and years after ICD implantation is crucial. Formal follow-up appointments are required about every 3 months to check that the device is functioning correctly and to assess battery life (Bleasdale et al. 2004). Given that inappropriate shocks can occur in about 12% of patients (Alter et al. 2005), it is important that the appropriateness of any ICD therapy be fully evaluated at follow-up.

One of the key aspects of caring for a patient after ICD implantation is consideration of the psychological and social impact of the procedure. Up to 38% of patients may suffer from a clinical anxiety disorder after implantation, linked to the impact of receiving ICD shocks and/or having a life-threatening condition (Sears and Conti 2002). ICD patients should be offered a multidisciplinary and individualised programme of education and support. Some clinical areas will recruit ICD patients into structured cardiac rehabilitation programmes, which may be beneficial in reducing anxiety and increasing physical activity (Fitchet et al. 2003).

Patients should be informed that they may lose consciousness before or during a shock, and family members should be reassured that there is no danger inherent in touching the patient during a shock (James 2002). Concern for the well-being of a partner may restrict sexual activity, and a patient should be reassured that, in the unlikely event of shock delivery during sex, the partner will not be harmed (James 2002). Contact numbers for specialist clinics or cardiac units should be provided so that patients can seek advice after the delivery of shocks, and many support groups exist to provide peer support and education.

One of the coping strategies often used by patients after ICD implantation is deliberate restriction of everyday activities in an attempt to prevent the occurrence of arrhythmias that require a shock (Sears and Conti 2002). It is important to reinforce to patients that most activities can be carried out as before, although some lifestyle modification may be necessary. The risks of sporting activity for ICD patients are unclear. Although shock delivery is not uncommon during sports, there is no evidence that this causes significant harm to patients (Lampert et al. 2006). Advice on sporting activity may therefore vary between clinicians, although there is a majority view that contact sports should be avoided (Lampert et al. 2006). For all patients, precautions should be taken around sources of electromagnetic interference as with permanent pacemakers (see above).

One major influence on lifestyle is that driving is forbidden for 6 months after ICD implantation, and may recommence only if no shocks have been delivered in the previous 6 months (Driving and Vehicles Licensing Agency or DVLA 2005). However, despite restrictions on driving, most patients of working age do return to employment after ICD implantation (Sears and Conti 2002).

CONCLUSION

The number of interventional cardiology procedures continues to rise year on year. Technology continues to develop, and procedures are continually refined to provide therapy for patients with CHD, heart failure and arrhythmias. For the healthcare practitioner, the challenge is to remain up to date with the latest developments, so that they can deliver care that is comprehensive, holistic and evidence-based.

REFERENCES

Alter P, Waldhans S, Plachta E, Moosdorf R, Grimm W (2005) Complications of implantable cardioverter defibrillator therapy in 440 consecutive patients. *Pacing and Clinical Electrophysiology* **28**: 926–32.

Archbold R, Robinson N, Schilling R (2004) Radial artery access for coronary angiography and percutaneous coronary intervention. *British Medical Journal* **329**: 443–6.

Barnett M (2002) Care of patients requiring cardiac pacing. In: Hatchett R, Thompson D (eds), *Cardiac Nursing. A comprehensive guide*. Edinburgh: Churchill Livingstone.

Bashore T, Bates E, Berger P et al. (2001) Cardiac catheterization laboratory standards: a report of the American College of Cardiology task force on clinical expert consensus documents (ACC/SCA&I committee to develop an expert consensus document on cardiac catheterisation laboratory standards). *Journal of the American College of Cardiology* **37**: 2170–214.

Betts T (2003) Regional survey of temporary transvenous pacing procedures and complications. *Postgraduate Medical Journal* **79**: 463–6.

Blancher S, Main C (2000) Cardiac Electrophysiology Procedures. In: Woods S, Froelicher E, Motzer S (eds), *Cardiac Nursing*, 4th edn. Philadelphia: Lippincott.

Bleasdale R, Frenneaux M (2004) Cardiac resynchronisation therapy: when the drugs don't work. *Heart* **90**(suppl VI): 2–4.

Bleasdale R, Ruskin J, O'Callaghan P (2004) The implantable cardioverter defibrillator. In: Fuster V, Wayne Alexander R, O'Rourke R (eds), *Hurst's The Heart*, 11th edn. New York: McGraw-Hill.

British Cardiovascular Intervention Society (2005) *BCIS Audit Returns: Adult Interventional Procedures Jan 2004 to Dec 2004*. Available from www.bcis.org.uk.

Busch M, Juel R, Newton K (2000) Cardiac catheterization. In: Woods S, Froelicher E, Motzer S (eds), *Cardiac Nursing*, 4th edn. Philadelphia: Lippincott.

Cunningham A (2005) *Report for European Heart Rhythm Association 2004*. Available from www.icservices.nhs.uk/ncasp/pages/audit_topics/CHD/AnnualReport2004.pdf

Dawkins K, Gershlick T, de Belder M et al. and Joint Working Group on Percutaneous Coronary Intervention of the British Cardiovascular Intervention Society and the British Cardiac Society (2005) Percutaneous coronary intervention: recommendations for good practice and training. *Heart* **91**(suppl VI): 1–27.

Department of Health (2000) *National Service Framework for Coronary Heart Disease*. London: Department of Health.

Department of Health (2005) *Leading the Way – Progress Report 2005*. London: Department of Health.

Driving and Vehicles Licensing Agency (2005) *At a Glance Guide to the Current Medical Standards of Fitness to Drive.* Available from www.dvla.gov.uk/at_a_glance/ch2_cardiovascular.htm

Dukkipati S, O'Neill W, Harjai K et al. (2004) Characteristics of cerebrovascular accidents after percutaneous coronary interventions. *Journal of the American College of Cardiology* **43**: 1161–7.

Fitchet A, Doherty P, Bundy C et al. (2003) Comprehensive cardiac rehabilitation programme for implantable cardioverter-defibrillator patients: a randomised controlled trial. *Heart* **89**: 155–60.

Gammage M (2000) Temporary cardiac pacing. *Heart* **83**: 715–20.

Grech E (2004a) Pathophysiology and investigation of coronary artery disease. In: Grech E (ed.), *ABC of Interventional Cardiology*. London: BMJ Publishing Group, pp 1–4.

Grech E (2004b) Non-coronary percutaneous intervention. In: Grech E (ed.), *ABC of Interventional Cardiology*. London: BMJ Publishing Group, pp 29–32.

Gregoratos G, Abrams J, Epstein A et al. (2002) *ACC/AHA/NASPE 2002 Guideline Update for Implantation of Cardiac Pacemakers and Antiarrhythmia Devices: A Report of the American College of Cardiology/American Heart Association Task Force on Practice Guidelines (ACC/AHA/NASPE Committee on Pacemaker Implantation)*. Available from www.acc.org/clinical/guidelines/pacemaker/pacemaker.pdf

Houghton T, Kaye G (2004) Implantable devices for treating tachyarrhythmias. In: Grech E (ed.), *ABC of Interventional Cardiology*. London: BMJ Publishing Group.

Inwood H (2002) *Adult Cardiac Surgery. Nursing care and management*. London: Whurr Publishers.

Jacobson C, Gerity D (2000) Pacemakers and implantable defibrillators. In: Woods S, Froelicher E, Motzer S (eds), *Cardiac Nursing*, 4th edn. Philadelphia: Lippincott.

James J (2002) Management and support of patients with internal cardioverter defibrillators. In: Hatchett R, Thompson D (eds), *Cardiac Nursing. A comprehensive guide*. Edinburgh: Churchill Livingstone.

Kaye G (2004) Percutaneous interventional electrophysiology. In: Grech E (ed.), *ABC of Interventional Cardiology*. London: BMJ Publishing Group, pp 37–40.

Kelly R, Steinhubl S (2005) Changing roles of anticoagulant and antiplatelet treatment during percutaneous coronary intervention. *Heart* **91**(suppl III): 16–19.

Lampert R, Cannom D, Olshansky B (2006) Safety of sports participation in patients with implantable cardioverter defibrillators: A survey of Heart Rhythm Society members. *Journal of Cardiovascular Electrophysiology* **17**: 11–15.

National Institute for Clinical Excellence (2004) *Balloon Valvuloplasty for Aortic Valve Stenosis in Adults and Children. Interventional Procedure Guidance 78.* London, NICE.

National Institute for Health and Clinical Excellence (2006) *Implantable Cardioverter Defibrillators for Arrhythmias. Review of Technology Appraisal 11*. London: NICE.

Pavia S, Wilkoff B (2001) The management of surgical complications of pacemaker and implantable cardioverter-defibrillators. *Current Opinion in Cardiology* **16**: 66–71.

Philipp R, Grech E (2004) Interventional pharmacotherapy. In: Grech E (ed.), *ABC of Interventional Cardiology*. London: BMJ Publishing Group, pp 25–8.

Piéchaud J (2004) Closing down: Transcatheter closure of intracardiac defects and vessel embolisations. *Heart* **90**: 1505–10.

Pollard S, Munks K, Wales C et al. 2003) Position and mobilisation post-angiography study (PAMPAS): a comparison of 4.5 hours and 2.5 hours bed rest. *Heart* **89**: 447–8.

Sears S, Conti J (2002) Quality of life and psychological functioning of ICD patients. *Heart* **87**: 488–93.

Silber S, Albertsson P, Avilés F, et al. (2005) European Society of Cardiology Guidelines for Percutaneous Coronary Interventions. *European Heart Journal* **26**: 804–47.

Vahanian A (2001) Balloon valvuloplasty. *Heart* **85**: 223–8.

Vahanian A, Palacios I (2004) Percutaneous approaches to Valvular disease. *Circulation* **109**: 1572–9.

Vijayaraman P, Ellenbogen K (2004) Bradyarrhythmias and pacemakers. In: Fuster V, Wayne Alexander R, O'Rourke R (eds), *Hurst's The Heart*, 11th edn. New York: McGraw-Hill.

Walsh K (2004) Interventional paediatric cardiology. In: Grech E (ed.), *ABC of Interventional Cardiology*. London: BMJ Publishing Group, pp 45–8.

West R, Ellis G, Brooks N (2005) Complications of diagnostic cardiac catheterisation: results from a confidential enquiry into cardiac catheter complications. *Heart* published online 24 Nov 2005 (doi: 10.1136/hrt.2005.073890).

Wiegand U, LeJeune D, Boguschewski F et al. (2004) Pocket hematoma after pacemaker or implantable cardioverter defibrillator surgery. *Chest* **126**: 1177–86.

Windecker S, Meier B (2000) Intervention in coronary artery disease. *Heart* **83**: 481–90.

15 Cardiac surgery

DIANE BURLEY and DAVID BARRETT

This chapter reviews the most commonly performed cardiac surgical procedures, focusing on indications for surgery and specific techniques. There is a discussion of the fundamentals of cardiac surgery in terms of pre-, peri- and postoperative care.

Much of the discussion focuses on coronary artery bypass (CAB) surgery, because this represents by far the most common cardiac surgical procedure. In 2002–3, almost 29 000 CAB operations were carried out in the UK – four times the number performed 20 years earlier (British Heart Foundation or BHF 2005). Surgery on diseased heart valves accounted for about 8500 operations in 2000–1, of which just under 3000 were performed in combination with CAB (Society of Cardiothoracic Surgeons of Great Britain and Ireland or SCTS 2002). Although other types of cardiac surgery are performed only rarely, they are discussed briefly, including heart transplantations, of which 219 were performed in 2000–1 – with 38 of these operations including lung transplantation (SCTS 2002).

TYPES OF CARDIAC SURGERY

CORONARY ARTERY BYPASS

CAB is an operation that provides symptom relief and improved prognosis for patients with coronary heart disease (CHD). It is most successful for patients with stable angina, who can be admitted for surgery electively. However, it can be used in emergencies as treatment for acute coronary syndromes.

Indications for CAB

Advances in percutaneous approaches to coronary revascularisation (see Chapter 14) have resulted in CAB generally being used in those patients with severe multi-vessel disease. Patients with left main stem stenosis may also be

Cardiac Care: An Introduction for Healthcare Professionals. Edited by David Barrett, Mark Gretton and Tom Quinn
© 2006 John Wiley & Sons Ltd

referred for CAB, given the potential risks of a percutaneous approach. Emergency CAB is usually carried out in patients with unstable multi-vessel disease not treatable with medication or percutaneous revascularisation, or in patients who have complications during coronary angioplasty.

Mortality rates

Mortality rates for CAB have fallen steadily over time. In 2002, the mortality rate for CAB operations in the UK was 1.8% (SCTS 2002). However, it should be recognised that mortality rates rise significantly in elderly patients, patients with existing co-morbidities and patients undergoing emergency surgery.

Surgical procedure

The surgery involves providing an alternative route for oxygenated blood to travel through the coronary circulation and perfuse the myocardium. Veins and arteries from the patient are used to bypass narrowed or obstructed sections of the native coronary arteries.

The most commonly used vein for CAB is the saphenous vein, which is removed from the leg ('harvested') at the beginning of surgery. During the procedure, one end of the harvested vein is joined to the aorta, just past the aortic valve. The other end of the vein is attached to the diseased coronary artery, just past the narrowed section, offering an alternative route for blood flow. Arteries can also be harvested and used in CAB. The radial artery is commonly used, and the same technique is used as with saphenous veins. In some patients, the internal mammary artery (IMA) is appropriate to use as an alternative route. As the IMA links directly to the aorta, it does not need to be completely excised from its normal position. Instead, one end of the IMA is detached and the free end brought down and joined to the narrowed coronary artery past the diseased section, thereby supplying oxygenated blood.

In the years after CAB, the grafts are susceptible to the same atherosclerotic disease process as the patient's native coronary arteries. If the grafts do become diseased, then the patient will become symptomatic and require 're-do' grafts using different veins and/or arteries. Re-do procedures are technically more difficult to perform and the mortality rates are therefore higher than in first-time operations. In terms of long-term function, arterial grafts are greatly superior to venous grafts. There is a body of evidence that suggests the use of IMAs instead of vein grafts results in long-term benefits such as less angina and a reduced chance of needing a re-do operation (Patil et al. 2001).

Specific postoperative care and rehabilitation

Patients undergoing CAB are often at high risk of suffering from reperfusion arrhythmias in the early postoperative period. Acute closure of the new grafts, usually caused by reduced perfusion or blood clot formation, is also a risk. For these reasons, close monitoring of the ECG is vital after CAB. A baseline 12-lead ECG should be obtained soon after return from theatre to assess the patient for ischaemia or infarction. This is particularly relevant where the IMA is used because arterial spasm can occur, leading to sudden ischaemic changes. In the days after surgery, any signs or symptoms of myocardial ischaemia must be assessed with an ECG and, if necessary, coronary angiography. Routine measurement of cardiac biomarkers to assess for myocardial infarction is of limited value because the trauma of heart surgery will usually result in marker release (Bojar 2005).

Secondary prevention of coronary events is an important element of recovery and rehabilitation in the patient after CAB. Unless contraindicated, patients should be discharged home on aspirin, a β blocker and a statin (Department of Health or DH 2000). Patients should also be supported in making lifestyle changes such as smoking cessation and increased exercise, to prevent further cardiac events. A fuller exploration of secondary prevention measures can be found in Chapter 3.

VALVE REPLACEMENT/REPAIR

Indications

Patients will usually be referred for valve surgery because of either stenosis or regurgitation, although infective endocarditis is another relatively common indication. The pathophysiology and presentation of valve disease are discussed in depth in Chapter 12. The vast majority of valve surgery is carried out on the mitral or aortic valve, although procedures are less commonly performed on the tricuspid valve.

A number of preoperative investigations, such as cardiac catheterisation and echocardiography, will be carried out to establish the severity of disease. Transoesophageal echocardiography (TOE) provides detailed information about valve function, and will often be used preoperatively, and sometimes perioperatively, as an assessment tool. These investigations may allow the surgeon to decide preoperatively whether to repair or to replace the valve, although the decision may be made intraoperatively. In general, valve repair is more likely to be performed when the disease process is at a less advanced stage (Lynn-McHale 2003).

Mortality rates

Valve operations are often carried out in combination with CAB, and in these cases mortality rates were 7.8% in 2000–1 (SCTS 2002). Valve operations carried out in isolation had an overall mortality rate of 4.8% in 2000–1 (SCTS

2002), although this varies considerably from patient to patient depending on risk profile and type of operation.

Surgical procedure

Valve repair

A number of different techniques can be used to repair a diseased valve, depending on the underlying disease process. If necessary, repairs can be made to the ring-shaped structure that supports the valve (annulus). These repairs can involve suturing the annulus to correct any deformities, or alternatively a prosthetic structure called an annuloplasty ring can be sewn into the valve to support the structure. If a valve is stenotic, a procedure called a commissurotomy is an option. In this, an incision is made down the valve margins that have become fused together. This incision should allow the valve leaflets to move freely again and the valve to open fully. Less commonly used methods of valve repair are required when valve dysfunction is caused by problems with the chordae tendineae or papillary muscle. The chordae tendineae can be repaired with sutures if they become detached or stretched. Papillary muscles, which can rupture as a complication of myocardial ischaemia or infarction, can also be repaired surgically.

Valve replacement

If a valve needs replacing, a decision is made whether to use a mechanical or a biological prosthetic valve (from a pig or human donor). This decision should be made preoperatively between the surgeon and the patient because the choice has long-term consequences. Patients who have mechanical valves implanted will need to be anticoagulated for the rest of their lives. This reliance on anticoagulants, and the resulting risks of excessive bleeding, may significantly affect the quality of life for individual patients. Patients who are at inherent risk of bleeding – such as elderly people – may therefore be best suited to a bioprosthetic valve where anticoagulation may not be necessary.

Another element of the decision-making process is the long-term function of the prosthetic valve. Biological prosthetic valves are likely to become dysfunctional and require replacement sooner than mechanical valves (Bloomfield 2002). For this reason, patients who are young at the time of valve replacement may prefer a mechanical valve because this is likely to need replacing less often during their lifetime. Conversely, a patient whose lifespan is expected to be relatively short (such as an octogenarian) may be more suited to a bioprosthetic valve, which should remain functional for the rest of his or her life (Pretre and Turina 2000).

During surgery, the diseased valve is removed and the prosthesis implanted. In the case of aortic valve replacement, it may also be necessary to replace the aortic root with a surgical graft (Bojar 2005).

Specific postoperative care and rehabilitation

Anticoagulation

Once the risk of immediate postoperative bleeding has passed, anticoagulation must be considered for patients after valve replacement. In the first few days postoperatively, heparin can be used to anticoagulate the patient, with warfarin used in the medium to long term. As previously mentioned, patients with mechanical valves will require anticoagulation for the rest of their lives. Although specific levels are dependent on the type of mechanical valve used and the valve(s) replaced, the target range for the international normalised ratio (INR) will usually be between 2.0 and 3.5 (Bojar 2005).

Patients who have bioprosthetic valves implanted will often be anticoagulated for up to 3 months after the operation (Salem et al. 2004). The target INR during this time is recommended as 2.5 (Salem et al. 2004). Patients with bioprosthetic valves who are considered to be at high risk of thromboembolic events (such as patients in atrial fibrillation), anticoagulation must be continued indefinitely. For patients at low risk of thrombus formation, long-term antiplatelet treatment with aspirin alone should be sufficient (Salem et al. 2004).

All patients who are receiving anticoagulation therapy are at risk of bleeding complications. Patients should therefore be educated about bleeding risks, and be encouraged to adapt their lifestyle accordingly (e.g. reducing or ceasing participation in contact sports).

Endocarditis

Mechanical and biological valves can be susceptible to endocarditis. For this reason, patients who require certain procedures (notably dental care) may require antibiotic prophylaxis to reduce their risks (Horstkotte et al. 2004). More information about endocarditis can be found in Chapter 12.

REPAIR OF STRUCTURAL DEFECTS

There are a number of surgical techniques for repairing structural cardiac defects. These defects can result either from congenital heart disease or from trauma or myocardial infarction (MI).

Septal defect repair

Atrial and ventricular septal defects can be closed percutaneously (see Chapter 14) or surgically. In general, percutaneous methods are used for atrial defects, whereas patients with ventricular defects are currently more likely to undergo surgical repair. Once the heart has been opened and the defect visualised, a patch is used to close the hole and prevent movement of blood between chambers.

Left ventricular aneurysm repair

Left ventricular aneurysms most commonly occur as a result of an MI causing thinning of one section of the myocardium. They can lead to heart failure, arrhythmias and thromboembolic events. Surgical repair of an aneurysm involves opening up the thinned myocardium, removing some if necessary, and then suturing and patching the ventricle (Bojar 2005).

Repair of the aorta

The aorta may require repair because of either aneurysm or dissection of the vessel wall. In both cases, the aorta may be repaired surgically, or the affected part of the vessel may need to be removed and replaced with a surgical graft (Bojar 2005).

Surgical interventions for heart failure

Left ventricular remodelling

At the end of the twentieth century there was great interest in the use of a surgical procedure called partial left ventriculectomy. This operation was designed for patients with severe heart failure, and involved resecting part of left ventricle. This would reduce the size of the left ventricle and improve the power of cardiac contractions (Acker 2004). However, disappointing medium- to long-term results of the operation have resulted in the popularity of this intervention declining (Acker 2004).

A number of different surgical interventions are currently being studied to evaluate their effectiveness. These include operations similar to that described for correcting left ventricular aneurysms, and the implantation of devices that physically shape or support the heart (Acker 2004).

Cardiac transplantation

Transplantation of the dysfunctional heart with a donor organ is the gold standard surgical therapy for patients with end-stage cardiac failure (Acker 2004). However, limited availability of donor organs means that this intervention is restricted to very few patients (Frazier and Delgado 2003).

Patients referred by their cardiologist for transplantation require a comprehensive transplant evaluation, which will provide an assessment of their overall state of health (Deng 2002). If the patient meets the strict criteria for acceptance, then he or she will be put onto the waiting list. Once on the active waiting list, patients may be called at any time if a suitable donor heart becomes available. Suitability of an organ for a particular patient is dependent on the donor having the same ABO blood type, and being of a similar weight (within 30%) as the recipient (Bethea et al. 2003).

The surgical procedure involves most, or all, of the recipient's heart being removed and the donor heart being implanted. One of the greatest risks of cardiac transplantation is rejection of the donor organ by the recipient. The risk of rejection is controlled by lifelong use of immunosuppressant drugs such as ciclosporin. Immunosuppressant drugs themselves cause problems – notably increasing the risk of opportunistic infections and of cancer in later life (Bethea et al. 2003).

Implantation of mechanical circulatory support

Patients who have severe heart failure or need temporary cardiac support (e.g. after cardiac surgery) may benefit from mechanical circulatory support (MCS). There are different types of device, providing support to either or both of the ventricles. In patients with end-stage heart failure, a left ventricular assist device (LVAD) may be indicated. LVADs are surgically implanted into the left ventricle and enhance systemic blood flow while reducing left ventricular workload. In the past, LVADs were used as a temporary measure while patients waited for transplantation (Frazier and Delgado 2003). However, patients who have received LVADs as an interim measure have demonstrated long-term improvement that has removed the need for transplantation (Frazier and Delgado 2003).

Long-term support of patients with implanted LVADs, leading to eventual recovery of left ventricular function, may therefore become more common in the future. As with any prosthetic implant, the risks of infection and thromboembolism are high, and most LVADs require patients to remain anticoagulated with warfarin (Kukuy et al. 2003).

FUNDAMENTALS OF CARDIAC SURGERY

PREOPERATIVE CARE

Most cardiac operations can be performed either electively or as emergency cases, and the preparation of patients will differ to some degree.

Preoperative assessment

Ideally, patients requiring cardiac surgery will be seen in a preoperative clinic, where informed consent can be gained and a full risk assessment carried out. A number of risk assessment tools are commonly used for patients before surgery. These allow the surgical team to weigh up the risks and benefits of performing the operation, and give the patient an individualised and objective measure of the possible dangers. Two commonly used scoring systems for cardiac patients are the Parsonnet score and the EuroScore. Although they differ in their calculations, they both consider those elements of a patient history that add to the risk of an operation, e.g. age, general health and type of operation.

In addition to a general risk assessment, there will also be assessment of any pre-existing renal, neurological, respiratory or endocrine disorders (particularly diabetes). Blood tests should be performed a few weeks before surgery, and on the day before the operation. There should be biochemical assessment of renal function, accompanied by a clotting screen and full blood count. In addition, the patient will often need a number of units of blood cross-matching before surgery.

Preparation for surgery

Any medication that the patient takes before surgery will be reviewed during the preoperative assessment. Exact policies on the discontinuation of medication will often vary depending on the preferences of the surgeon performing the operation. However, as a general rule, most cardiac drugs such as β blockers, nitrates and anti-arrhythmic agents are continued up to and including the day of surgery. Any patients taking hormone replacement therapy or an oral contraceptive should stop these in the weeks running up to surgery because they can increase the risk of venous thrombosis (Eagle et al. 2004).

Anticoagulant and antiplatelet medications need to be managed carefully before cardiac surgery. Warfarin should be stopped a few days before surgery, with many surgeons unwilling to operate until the INR is within certain, locally determined, limits. If patients are considered at risk of thrombotic events before surgery, then anticoagulation can be achieved by treatment with heparin, the effects of which can be easily reversed during surgery by giving protamine. In cases of extreme emergencies, surgery may go ahead when anticoagulants have not been stopped. In these cases, the patient will be given platelets and freshly frozen plasma (FFP) to try to normalise clotting levels. Some surgeons may allow patients to take aspirin up until the day of surgery, whereas others prefer all antiplatelet therapy to stop. The increasing use of clopidogrel as an antiplatelet for patients with acute coronary syndromes has implications for those requiring cardiac surgery. Receiving clopidogrel in the days before cardiac surgery significantly increases the risk of peri- and postoperative bleeding (Kapetanakis et al. 2005). Local policies should therefore include guidance on when and how patients are informed to stop clopidogrel.

The requirements of the preoperative shave will often vary between surgical units. However, female patients rarely require any hair removal before cardiac surgery. Men will generally need their chest shaving, along with any other areas that may require surgical incision, e.g. the legs in the case of a patient having CAB. Patients are generally required to fast for 4–6 hours before cardiac surgery, with clear fluids allowed up to 2 hours before the start of surgery (Inwood 2002). Where fasting times are longer as a result of a delay in start times, intravenous fluids should be considered to prevent dehydration.

The content and timing of pre-medication will vary according to local policy. However, most patients will be given a sedative a few hours before surgery and continuous oxygen therapy will be commenced (Inwood 2002).

PERIOPERATIVE CARE

Wound site

For most types of cardiac surgery, access to the heart is through a sternal wound called a median sternotomy. After a skin incision is made, the sternum is split with an air-driven saw. After surgery, the sternum is wired together using sternal wire and the skin sutured. The wound will then be covered with a sterile dressing for 24–48 hours postoperatively.

In some cases, the surgeon may deem it undesirable to close the wound immediately after surgery, e.g. if the patient is at particular risk of internal haemorrhage or if the heart has become abnormally dilated during surgery. In these cases, the patient's sternal wound will be packed and covered with a sterile dressing until closure is carried out, although specific wound care will vary between surgeons.

Techniques have been developed that allow cardiac surgery to be performed using a minimally invasive approach. Minimally invasive techniques have been used in patients requiring CAB only to the left anterior descending (LAD) coronary artery – an operation called minimally invasive direct coronary artery bypass (MIDCAB) (Bojar 2005). Instead of a sternotomy, the surgery is carried out through an incision in the fourth or fifth intercostal space on the left side of the chest. Although simpler than CAB involving a sternotomy, a recent review of MIDCAB in the UK did not find any evidence that the technique was more effective than percutaneous angioplasty in the treatment of LAD disease (Reeves et al. 2004). For this reason, the use of MIDCAB may remain relatively limited.

Cardiopulmonary bypass

The complexities of cardiac surgery mean that many operations require the heart to be stopped, with no blood present in the surgical field. When required, this is achieved through the establishment of cardiopulmonary bypass (CPB).

The inferior and superior venae cavae are cannulated, and venous blood drained into the bypass machine, which comprises an oxygenator and pump. The venous blood is oxygenated, anticoagulated with heparin to prevent thrombosis, and pumped back into the patient's systemic circulation via the aorta. Once CPB is established, cardiac function is stopped (cardioplegia) by the insertion of a potassium-rich solution into the heart and coronary arteries. Cardioplegia solution will be infused every 20 minutes during surgery to maintain cardiac arrest. The cardioplegia solution used to stop the heart can also protect the myocardium from the effects of minimal perfusion of blood during surgery. This solution is often cold, slowing the metabolic rate of myocardial cells, thereby reducing oxygen demand and decreasing the likelihood of ischaemia or infarction. Once surgery is completed, the effects of the cardioplegia solution are allowed to wear off, and the heart begins to fibrillate. Normal cardiac function is then restored through defibrillation with internal paddles.

Although CPB is essential for many cardiac surgical procedures, it does have a number of drawbacks. The passage of blood against the internal surfaces of the bypass machine causes a systemic inflammatory response and the production of emboli. These can, in turn, lead to clotting disorders and damage to the heart, kidneys and brain (Murphy et al. 2004).

As a result of the potential complications of CPB, there is increasing interest in carrying out cardiac surgery while the heart is still beating. So-called 'off-pump' surgery is particularly applicable for patients requiring CAB, where it has been shown to result in fewer short-term complications than surgery using CPB (Murphy et al. 2004). Long-term studies are ongoing to explore whether grafts attached during off-pump CAB maintain the patency of traditionally attached grafts over a period of years. Pending the results from these studies, it seems likely that off-pump CAB will continue to grow in popularity as a surgical technique.

POSTOPERATIVE CARE

Most patients require care in either an intensive care (ICU) or high dependency (HDU) area immediately after surgery. This is to expedite recovery times and to detect and treat complications effectively.

Respiratory care and complications

Most patients leave the operating theatre with an endotracheal tube (ET) *in situ* and mechanical ventilation ongoing. Arterial blood gases (ABGs) are taken regularly to ensure that ventilation is providing optimum oxygen delivery and the removal of carbon dioxide. Mechanical ventilation allows a period of stability until the possibility of postoperative complications has been minimised. However, it is one of the goals within the ICU to promote spontaneous breathing as quickly as possible, although the ability to achieve this may be affected by underlying lung disease or the occurrence of peri- or postoperative complications (Bojar 2005).

Different post-surgical units will have different policies for weaning patients off mechanical ventilation and removing the ET tube (extubation). Generally, signs that the patient is ready for weaning are either signs of wakefulness or an increasing number of spontaneous breaths being taken (Inwood 2002). When weaning is deemed appropriate, the input of mechanical ventilation is slowly decreased, resulting in the patient taking increased responsibility for breathing. Progress is monitored through pulse oximetry and ABG measurement. Extubation is indicated once the patient is breathing spontaneously, is able to follow commands and demonstrates a strong cough or gag reflex.

Cardiovascular care and complications

Arrhythmias

All patients will require a period of cardiac monitoring after surgery as a result of the high incidence of arrhythmias. Atrial fibrillation (AF) is one of the most common post-surgical complications – occurring in about 30% of patients after CAB (Eagle et al. 2004). Although AF will increase the length of hospital stay, the priority is the recognition and prompt treatment of life-threatening arrhythmias such as ventricular fibrillation, ventricular tachycardia and complete heart block. Patients with cardiac arrest or peri-arrest rhythms such as these should be given emergency treatment as discussed in Chapter 10.

Some prophylactic steps can be taken to prevent the likelihood of arrhythmias. The administration of β blockers postoperatively has been shown to lower the risk of AF occurring (Bojar 2005). More recently, a surgical procedure to prevent AF – the 'Maze' procedure – has become more commonplace. The Maze procedure involves making small surgical incisions within the atria to interrupt any re-entry circuits that may cause AF (Earley and Schilling 2006).

To counter the risk of bradyarrhythmias, many patients will be fitted with pacing wires during surgery; known as epicardial wires, they are fixed directly into the outer wall of the right atrium or ventricle. Although they may not be required, the wires are left *in situ* postoperatively, with the other end of the wires outside the chest wall. Connection to a temporary pacemaker box can therefore be quickly achieved in the event of the patient becoming bradycardic. Epicardial pacing wires are often left in place until day 4 or 5 postoperatively, after which, if the patient shows no signs of developing heart block, they can be removed. Their removal can, in itself, cause complications such as haemorrhage and/or cardiac tamponade. Therefore, local policies will be in place outlining criteria for clotting results before the removal of pacing wires. Only practitioners with the appropriate training should carry out the procedure, and patients should be observed closely for at least 1 hour afterwards.

Haemorrhage and fluid replacement

Careful fluid management is required in the hours following cardiac surgery, because external and internal haemorrhage is a significant risk. This is usually done with colloid replacement in the form of blood and blood products, although each clinical area should have local guidelines for fluid management. A multi-lumen catheter is usually inserted into either the subclavian or internal jugular vein on induction of anaesthesia. This facilitates the monitoring of central venous pressure (CVP) and administration of fluids, and offers direct access for intravenous medication. Having access into a large vein allows strong concentrations of drugs to be given quickly and effectively, as is necessary in emergency situations.

In some patients, bleeding will occur into the pericardial space. If bleeding into the pericardial space continues, pressure will rise and the heart become constricted. This is a condition known as cardiac tamponade. Cardiac tamponade presents with signs and symptoms representative of reduced cardiac output, such as hypotension, tachycardia, raised CVP and low urine output. If left uncorrected, cardiac tamponade will lead to a progressive decrease in cardiac function, culminating in cardiac arrest. This can be either a gradual process or happen very suddenly. Cardiac tamponade usually warrants a further surgical procedure to evacuate the collection of blood and identify the bleeding point (Bojar 2005).

To reduce the risk of tamponade, and monitor for internal haemorrhage, patients will return from surgery with a number of chest drains inserted. Blood loss through the drains must be observed closely in the postoperative period to monitor for haemorrhage and ensure drain patency. Patients with excessive blood loss may need fluid replacement with colloids or blood, additional reversal of the effects of heparin or even a return to the operating theatre (Inwood 2002).

Re-warming

The long period of time spent in the operating theatre, coupled with an open chest cavity, and the cooling effects of CPB, will usually cause a systemic hypothermia (Withers 2005).

Much of the initial re-warming is carried out using CPB while the patient is still in the operating theatre. However, many patients will arrive in the critical care setting postoperatively with a core temperature of between 34 and 35°C (Bojar 2005). A number of different re-warming strategies can be utilised postoperatively. The patient may be externally warmed using passive methods such as blankets, or active methods including blankets with warm air circulating within them. Re-warming of the patient after cardiac surgery brings with it a number of risks. If re-warming is too rapid, peripheral vasodilatation can occur, causing a sudden drop in blood pressure. It is also possible that too rapid re-warming could cause the patient to become pyrexial. For this reason, active re-warming should be discontinued once the patient's temperature reaches 36.4°C (Inwood 2002).

Alterations in cardiac output

Arrhythmias, haemorrhage and re-warming can all cause hypotension after cardiac surgery. In addition, hypotension may be caused by impaired contractility of cardiac muscle after surgery. In many patients, the functional capability of cardiac muscle will be impaired for 6–8 hours after surgery. In an uncomplicated patient, myocardial function will return to preoperative levels within about 24 hours (Bojar 2005).

A number of patients may be hypertensive after cardiac surgery. This is often the result of a sympathetic nervous system response to the use of cardiopulmonary bypass and the surgery itself. Hypertension after surgery presents a number of risks, notably the increased likelihood of bleeding (Inwood 2002).

The patient's cardiac function will be closely monitored for at least 24 hours. An arterial line should be inserted to provide continuous blood pressure monitoring. Many critical care areas will also use a pulmonary artery (PA) catheter, to provide an assessment of left ventricular function.

Impaired myocardial function can be supported pharmacologically or mechanically. Inotropic agents such as dopamine, dobutamine, adrenaline (epinephrine) and noradrenaline (norepinephrine) can be infused to improve contractility of the heart (see Chapter 13). Patients with impaired cardiac function can also be assisted through the initiation of intra-aortic balloon counterpulsation (IABC). IABC is used to lessen the workload of the left ventricle and to increase perfusion of the coronary arteries.

Thromboembolic events

As with any operation, patients undergoing cardiac surgery are at risk of suffering thromboembolic events such as deep vein thrombosis (DVT) and/or pulmonary embolism (PE). Three standard prophylactic measures can be taken to reduce the incidence of DVT/PE.

First, by mobilising early and exercising the leg muscles, patients can greatly reduce their chances of developing a DVT. Patients should be encouraged to start mobilising as soon as is clinically appropriate after surgery. If possible, this mobilisation should consist of at least 5 minutes of walking each hour (Inwood 2002). Patients should also be fitted with anti-embolism stockings. By compressing the legs, anti-embolism stockings improve venous flow and reduce the likelihood of clots forming. Knee-length and thigh-length stockings are available, and the patient's legs must be measured each morning to ensure that the correct size stockings are applied. Finally, low-molecular-weight heparin (LMWH), administered subcutaneously, is an effective pharmacological agent in the prevention of thromboembolic events. In each patient, the benefits of heparin prophylaxis will have to be balanced against the potential risk of bleeding from wound sites.

Neurological care

Most patients will return from cardiac surgery with their cognitive function still dulled by anaesthesia and continuing sedation. This makes the assessment of neurological function difficult in the early postoperative phase. While the patient remains ventilated, some level of sedation will usually be required. However, patients should ideally be sedated to such a level that they can be roused by either voice or touch (Inwood 2002). Once sedation has been discontinued, a full neurological assessment of the patient should be carried out. The tool most commonly used for this assessment is the Glasgow Coma Scale (GCS), which provides information about eye opening, motor response and verbal response.

The most damaging neurological complication after cardiac surgery is a cerebrovascular accident (CVA) or stroke. The risk of a stroke is about 2–6% after cardiac surgery, and is often related to either embolic events or significant hypotension during or after the operation (Pandit and Pigott 2001, Bojar 2005). Where a CVA is suspected as a result of impaired neurological function, a computed tomography (CT) scan should be performed to identify whether the incident is haemorrhagic or embolic in nature. If haemorrhage can be ruled out, anticoagulation therapy with heparin should be commenced (Bojar 2005).

Renal care

The kidneys receive about 25% of total cardiac output, and are therefore acutely sensitive to any haemodynamic instability. Overall, patients undergoing cardiac surgery have a 2% chance of developing renal failure postoperatively, but the incidence is greatly increased in patients with any history of kidney problems before surgery (Inwood 2002, Bojar 2005).

Renal function is monitored primarily through the hourly measurement of urine output in the immediate postoperative period. Should the urine output fall below approximately 0.5 ml/kg per hour, treatment should be instigated. Treatment would initially entail careful fluid management to enhance renal perfusion while avoiding fluid overload.

If the renal dysfunction is significant, and the patient loses the ability effectively to excrete electrolytes and waste products, renal replacement therapy (RRT) will be necessary. RRT in the context of critical care usually entails haemofiltration – a slow continuous process in which an artificial kidney filters the blood to remove waste products, solutes and excess fluid. This can be particularly valuable because it allows the patient's fluid balance to be manipulated and gives capacity to provide the patient with supportive drug therapy and, if necessary, an enteral feed.

Pain relief and wound care

After cardiac surgery, the main focus of pain is the sternal wound. However, additional wound sites (such as the leg in some CAB operations) can often cause greater discomfort in the days and weeks after surgery. In the immediate postoperative period, pain relief is usually achieved using intravenous opioid analgesics such as morphine, although regimes will vary depending on local policy. As the patient recovers from surgery, opioid analgesia can be supplemented and eventually replaced by non-steroidal anti-inflammatory drugs (NSAIDs) such as diclofenac. Some cardiac surgical centres will also use different approaches to providing pain relief postoperatively, such as epidural analgesia or patient-controlled analgesia in which the patient controls the administration of medication (Dawkins 2003).

After surgery, wound sites all present a risk of infection and intravenous antibiotics are given as prophylaxis to all patients during and after the operation. Deep sternal wound infection – mediastinitis – is a potentially fatal complication of cardiac surgery. It occurs in 1–4% of cases, and has a mortality rate of about 25% (Eagle et al. 2004). Wounds should be observed regularly to detect any signs of infection (e.g. redness, heat, pus) and swabs taken if necessary to identify the type of pathogen involved. Although antibiotic treatment is usually sufficient to treat minor infections, it is possible that some patients may require surgical débridement of infected tissue (Bojar 2005). In the days after surgery, patients should be encouraged to keep wounds clean and dry, with showers being preferable to baths for meeting hygiene needs. Patients should be educated about the signs of wound infection, and the use of simple analgesia when required should be encouraged for the first few weeks.

Rehabilitation

After common cardiac surgical procedures, most patients will spend about 5–7 days in hospital postoperatively. However, discharge home marks the beginning of a long period of rehabilitation guided in part by the healthcare team.

Education and counselling

Although cardiac surgery will usually bring about an improvement in wellbeing, it also presents a number of physical, social and psychological challenges for the patient to overcome. The period of recovery after cardiac surgery can also be a stressful time for the patient's family and carers. Efforts should therefore be made to include significant others in the rehabilitation of patients wherever possible.

The speed of recovery will vary from patient to patient; it may take at least 3 months to rehabilitate fully after major cardiac surgery. Patients will need to be educated about increasing their level of physical activity in the weeks and months after surgery. In the immediate post-discharge period, patients will feel very tired, but should try to carry out some limited exercise (e.g. short walks, light housework, climbing stairs) each day. More intense activity, such as lifting heavy loads, should be avoided for the first 2–3 months to avoid excessive strain on the heart and prevent damage to the healing sternal wound.

Many cardiac rehabilitation teams provide an exercise programme for patients who have had cardiac surgery. These allow patients to participate in a structured exercise routine under the supervision of healthcare staff for the first few weeks after discharge.

Many patients will wish to know when they can resume sexual activity. This is generally a decision that can be made by the patient and his or her partner. However, patients should be advised that care must be taken not to put pressure on the sternum in the first few months after surgery. Patients should be educated about the psychological effects of cardiac surgery along with the physical. Six months after cardiac surgery, 10–30% of patients still have some cognitive dysfunction (Pandit and Pigott 2001). A similar percentage will continue to experience psychological symptoms such as hallucinations for a number of months after cardiac surgery (Inwood 2002).

The length of time that a patient requires off work after surgery will depend greatly on the type of employment. Although most patients will require at least 6 weeks off work, this period will be significantly extended for a patient who has a physical job. Guidelines on how long patients must refrain from driving vary depending on the type of surgery undergone and the vehicle licence held. Patients should be referred to the guidance available from the Driving and Vehicle Licensing Agency (DVLA) at www.dvla.gov.uk.

CONCLUSION

Despite rapid developments in the pharmacological and percutaneous treatment of heart diseases, cardiac surgery remains an important treatment option. Although the bulk of cardiac surgery provides relief from the symptoms of CHD, patients with valve disorders, structural abnormalities or severe heart failure may also benefit. The role of the healthcare practitioner when caring for a patient undergoing cardiac surgery is to prepare and then guide him or her through the significant physical and psychological challenges posed by this major life event.

REFERENCES

Acker A (2004) Surgical therapies for heart failure. *Journal of Cardiac Failure* **10**: S220–4.

Bethea B, Yuh D, Conte J, Baumgartner WA (2003) Heart transplantation. In: Cohn LH, Edmunds LH Jr (eds), *Cardiac Surgery in the Adult*. New York: McGraw-Hill, pp 1427–60.

Bloomfield P (2002) Choice of heart valve prosthesis. *Heart* **87**: 583–9.

Bojar R (2005) *Manual of Perioperative Care in Cardiac Surgery*, 4th edn. Boston, MA: Blackwell Publishing.

British Heart Foundation (2005) *Coronary Heart Disease Statistics*. London: BHF.

Dawkins S (2003) Patient-controlled analgesia after coronary artery bypass grafting. *Nursing Times* **99**(47): 30–1.

Deng M (2002) Cardiac transplantation. *Heart* **87**: 177–84.

Department of Health (2000) *National Service Framework for Coronary Heart Disease*. London: Department of Health.

Eagle K, Guyton R, Davidoff R et al. (2004) *ACC/AHA 2004 guideline update for coronary artery bypass graft surgery: a report of the American College of Cardiology/ American Heart Association Task Force on Practice Guidelines*. Available from:http:// www.acc.org/clinical/guidelines/cabg/index.pdf

Earley M, Schilling R (2006) Catheter and surgical ablation of atrial fibrillation. *Heart* **92**: 266–74.

Frazier O, Delgado R (2003) Mechanical circulatory support for advanced heart failure. Where does it stand in 2003? *Circulation* **108**: 3064–8.

Horstkotte D, Follath F, Gutschik E et al. (2004) Guidelines on prevention, diagnosis and treatment of infective endocarditis. Executive summary. *European Heart Journal* **25**: 267–76.

Inwood H (2002) *Adult Cardiac Surgery: Nursing care and management* London: Whurr Publishers.

Kapetanakis E, Medlam D, Boyce S et al. (2005) Clopidogrel administration prior to coronary artery bypass grafting surgery: the cardiologist's panacea or the surgeon's headache? *European Heart Journal* **26**: 576–83.

Kukuy EL, Oz MC, Naka Y (2003) Long-term mechanical circulatory support. In: Cohn LH, Edmunds LH Jr (eds), *Cardiac Surgery in the Adult*. New York: McGraw-Hill, pp 1491–506.

Lynn-McHale D (2003) Advances in cardiac surgery: valve repair. *Critical Care Nurse* **23**(2): 72–87.

Murphy G, Ascione R, Angelini G (2004) Coronary artery bypass grafting on the beating heart: surgical revascularization for the next decade? *European Heart Journal* **25**: 2077–85.

Pandit J, Pigott D (2001) Cognitive dysfunction after cardiac surgery: strategies for prevention. *The British Journal of Cardiology* **8**: 613–16.

Patil C, Nikolsky E, Boulos E, Grenadier E, Beyar R (2001) Multivessel coronary artery disease: current revascularisation strategies. *European Heart Journal* **22**: 1183–97.

Pretre R, Turina M (2000) Cardiac valve surgery in the octogenarian. *Heart* **83**: 116–21.

Reeves B, Angelini G, Bryan A et al. (2004) A multi-centre randomised controlled trial of minimally invasive direct coronary bypass grafting versus percutaneous transluminal coronary angioplasty with stenting for proximal stenosis of the left anterior descending coronary artery. *Health Technology Assessment* **8**(16): 1–58.

Salem D, Stein P, Al-Ahmad A et al. (2004) Antithrombotic therapy in valvular heart disease – native and prosthetic. *Chest* **126**: 457S–82S.

Society of Cardiothoracic Surgeons of Great Britain and Ireland (2002) *National Adult Cardiac Surgical Database Report 2000–2001.* Available from www.scts.org

Withers J (2005) The elective re-warming of post-operative cardiac patients. *Nursing Standard* **101**(24): 30–3.

Index

Cardiac Care: An Introduction for Healthcare Professionals. Edited by David Barrett, Mark Gretton and Tom Quinn
© 2006 John Wiley & Sons Ltd